AF772866

NUTRITION AND DIET RESEARCH PROGRESS

DIETARY FIBER

PRODUCTION CHALLENGES, FOOD SOURCES AND HEALTH BENEFITS

NUTRITION AND DIET RESEARCH PROGRESS

Additional books in this series can be found on Nova's website
under the Series tab.

Additional e-books in this series can be found on Nova's website
under the e-book tab.

NUTRITION AND DIET RESEARCH PROGRESS

DIETARY FIBER

PRODUCTION CHALLENGES, FOOD SOURCES AND HEALTH BENEFITS

MARVIN E. CLEMENS
EDITOR

nova publishers
New York

Copyright © 2015 by Nova Science Publishers, Inc.

All rights reserved. No part of this book may be reproduced, stored in a retrieval system or transmitted in any form or by any means: electronic, electrostatic, magnetic, tape, mechanical photocopying, recording or otherwise without the written permission of the Publisher.

For permission to use material from this book please contact us:
nova.main@novapublishers.com

NOTICE TO THE READER

The Publisher has taken reasonable care in the preparation of this book, but makes no expressed or implied warranty of any kind and assumes no responsibility for any errors or omissions. No liability is assumed for incidental or consequential damages in connection with or arising out of information contained in this book. The Publisher shall not be liable for any special, consequential, or exemplary damages resulting, in whole or in part, from the readers' use of, or reliance upon, this material. Any parts of this book based on government reports are so indicated and copyright is claimed for those parts to the extent applicable to compilations of such works.

Independent verification should be sought for any data, advice or recommendations contained in this book. In addition, no responsibility is assumed by the publisher for any injury and/or damage to persons or property arising from any methods, products, instructions, ideas or otherwise contained in this publication.

This publication is designed to provide accurate and authoritative information with regard to the subject matter covered herein. It is sold with the clear understanding that the Publisher is not engaged in rendering legal or any other professional services. If legal or any other expert assistance is required, the services of a competent person should be sought. FROM A DECLARATION OF PARTICIPANTS JOINTLY ADOPTED BY A COMMITTEE OF THE AMERICAN BAR ASSOCIATION AND A COMMITTEE OF PUBLISHERS.

Additional color graphics may be available in the e-book version of this book.

Library of Congress Cataloging-in-Publication Data

ISBN: 978-1-63463-655-1

Library of Congress Control Number: 2014956991

Published by Nova Science Publishers, Inc. † New York

CONTENTS

PREFACE

Dietary fibers are classified into water soluble or insoluble, and most plant foods include in their composition variable amounts of a mixture of soluble and insoluble fibers. This soluble or insoluble nature of fiber is related to its physiological effects. Insoluble fibers are characterized by high porosity, low density and the ability to increase fecal bulk, and act by facilitating intestinal transit, thus reducing the exposure to carcinogens in the colon and therefore acting as protectors against colon cancer. The influence of soluble fiber in the digestive tract includes its ability to retain water and form gels as well as a role as a substrate for fermentation of colon bacteria. This book discusses the production challenges, food sources and health benefits of dietary fiber.

Chapter 1 - Starch is a polysaccharide abundant in nature that undergoes hydrolysis in the small intestine to provide energy in the form of glucose.

Portions of starch resistant to hydrolysis that escape the small intestine and enter the large intestine intact to undergo fermentation is known as resistant starch (RS). Fivetypes of RS, 1-5, have been identified based on the physical inaccessibility, structure, retrogradation, or chemical modification of starch found either naturally or added to food. Thus, RS can be classified as a dietary or functional fiber. The formulation of ingredients containing RS by the food industry, such as high-amylose maize, can increase the fiber content of food without altering physiochemical or sensory attributes. The small molecular size, bland flavor, and white color, make RS an ideal partial replacement for fully-digestible starch in food.

A reduction in caloric availability is observed when RS replaces fully-digestible starch and can attenuate postprandial glucose and insulin concentrations. Additional physiological effects of RS result from the production of short chain fatty acids upon fermentation in the large intestine. RS improves digestive health by acting as a prebiotic, decreasing intestinal pH, and the formation of cancer-causing agents.

In murine models, dietary RS is associated with reductions in total and abdominal adiposity and improvements in lean mass. Increases in intestinal-derived satiety hormones, such as peptide YY and glucagon-like peptide-1, contribute to these findings. Despite mixed results associated with changes in blood glucose and insulin concentrations after long-term RS consumption, adults consuming 15-40 g daily have shown improvements in insulin sensitivity, particularly among those with metabolic syndrome.

RS is a functional fiber that can increase dietary fiber intake and positively impact overall health when consumed in adequate amounts.

Chapter 2 - Dietary fibers are classified into water soluble or insoluble, and most plant foods include in their composition variable amounts of a mixture of soluble and insoluble fibers. This soluble or insoluble nature of fiber is related to its physiological effects. Insoluble fibers are characterized by high porosity, low density and the ability to increase fecal bulk, and act by facilitating intestinal transit, thus reducing the exposure to carcinogens in the colon and therefore acting as protectors against colon cancer. The influence of soluble fiber in the digestive tract includes its ability to retain water and form gels as well as a role as a substrate for fermentation of colon bacteria. However, the viscous soluble polysaccharides can delay digestion and compromise in some degree the absorption of nutrients from the gut.

Dietary fibers have an impact on all aspects of gut physiology and are a vital part of a healthy diet. Diets rich in dietary fiber have a protective effect against diseases such as hemorrhoids and some chronic diseases as well as in decreasing the incidence of various types of cancer, including colorectal, prostate and breast cancer.

The dietary fibers are among the most attractive and studied themes in nutrition and public health in the past decades, and therefore many epidemiological studies have been developed to evaluate the effects of fibers on several aspects of human health.

The current trend is towards diets rich in dietary fiber since these are implicated in the maintenance and/or improvement of health. However, despite the beneficial effects, there is also evidence of some negative effects associated with fiber consumption. For example, fiber can produce phytobenzoates, which can induce a decrease in the absorption and digestion of proteins. On the other hand, some fibers may inhibit the activity of pancreatic enzymes that digest carbohydrates, lipids and proteins. Furthermore, fibers can interfere, although not strongly, with the absorption of some vitamins and minerals like calcium, iron, zinc and copper.

Chapter 3 - The authors aimed to evaluate the effect of the prebiotics Nutriose® FB06 (NUT) and Raftilose® P95 (RAF) upon uptake of ^{14}C-butyrate (^{14}C-BT), and upon its cellular effects, in a rat normal intestinal epithelial cell line (IEC-6 cells). A long exposure (48h) to NUT or RAF (20-100 mg/ml) caused an increase in ^{14}C-BT uptake. This effect involved the sodium-dependent monocarboxylate transporter 1 (SMCT1) but not the proton-coupled monocarboxylate 1 transporter (MCT1), although prebiotics showed no effect on SMCT1 and MCT1 mRNA expression levels. BT (5 mM; 48h) markedly decreased cellular viability and culture growth and increased cell differentiation. Combination of prebiotics with BT did not significantly modify these parameters. In conclusion, the results show that a long exposure to NUT and RAF increases uptake of a low concentration of ^{14}C-BT by intestinal epithelial cells, although the prebiotics do not modify the effects of BT upon cell viability, culture growth and differentiation.

Chapter 4 - *Background:* It is thought that our genomic heritage from late Paleolithic man, 40,000 – 100,000 years ago, influenced not only our phenotype, but also our physiological functions. Our ancestors, for approximately 84,000 generations, survived on a regimen in which plants constituted from 50 to 80% of their diet. Later during the Neolithic agricultural period, our ancestors increased fiber intake even more to amounts that would have exceeded 100g/day. Thereafter, the industrial and agro business eras (200 years ago), and the digital age (2 generations ago) have distanced the nutrition from its primate and Paleolithic ancestors. It is known that fiber, and its sources, whole grain, fruits, and vegetables are also rich in minerals, vitamins, phenolic compounds, phytoestrogens, and related antioxidants. Thus, in conjunction with the discordance between our ancient genetically determined biology and the nutritional, cultural, and activity patterns in contemporary populations that adopted the "western lifestyle", many of the so-called disease of our time have emerged. Consumption of grain products milled from all edible components of grains, have been inversely associated with mortality from a number of chronic diseases.

Objective: To find the determinants of dietary fiber intake and its role in metabolic syndrome (MetS) in a community based intervention.

Design: It was a cross-sectional study of the relationship of ingested fibers with demographic, socieconomic, anthropometric, overall health perception, and specific pathognomonic markers for obesity and MetS and each of its components. The analysis came from baseline data obtained from participants of both sexes, over 35 years of age, enrolled during the 2007-2013 period (n= 605), in the ongoing dynamic cohort, Botucatu longitudinal study "Move for health" and conducted by professionals from the Nutritional and Exercise Metabolism Centre (CeMENutri) of the Botucatu Medical School (SP, Brazil).

Results: Even in the highest quartile, dietary fiber was far below the daily recommended intake, along with its source of fruits, vegetables, and whole grains. The quartile distribution of dietary fiber intake was not influenced by any of the study variables (demographic, socieconomic, anthropometric, overall health perception, or specific pathognomonic markers for obesity and MetS); however, in association-designed studies the authors had found that low dietary fiber intake and its sources represent a risk factor for insulin resistance, high-blood pressure and the presence of MetS. Moreover, in longitudinal studies with lifestyle changing (LISC) interventions, the authors noted a faster resolution of MetS when individuals met the recommended daily dietary fiber intake than only with LISC isolated.

Conclusion: Overall individuals had a high caloric diet and a low intake of all sources of fiber. These results were irrespective to age, gender, literacy and economic reasons, probably cultural, what makes the solution more difficult. However, when these subjects were enrolled in intervention programs with LISC it was found that adding dietary fiber to the diet was an effective booster for faster resolution of MetS. Therefore, the diet adequacy of fiber seems to work by diluting the energy intake that would potentiate the higher energy expenditure of physical exercise in promoting weight (body fat) loss, along with insulin sensitivity, vasodilation, lower inflammation states, etc.

Chapter 5 - The fiber fraction of plant cell walls is one of the major sources of nutrients and energy. Mammals do not produce enzymes that can hydrolyze β1-4 linked polysaccharides (cellulose and hemicellulose) of plant cell walls, and as such fiber cannot be directly used to feed the growing global human population. By symbiosis with rumen microbes, ruminants are capable of converting this non-digestible food resource into high-quality animal products. For dairy cows, fiber is an important feed component, not only as an energy and nutrient source, but also as a regulatory factor for the maintenance of rumen health and feed intake. Compared to other nutrients, fiber, particularly forage-fiber, has much longer ruminal retention time because of slower degradation and greater buoyancy in the rumen. As such feeding fiber with large particle size can increases digesta mass in the rumen that in turn stimulate rumination, increases rumen buffering capacity and reduces the risk of ruminal acidosis and abomasal displacement. On the other hand rumen-fill can also limit feed intake, and the filling effect of fiber in more pronounced in high producing dairy cows. Any reduction in dry matter intake reduces milk and milk protein yield of dairy cows. Therefore, high producing dairy cows can be benifited from feeding fiber sources with rapid rumen-passage rate.

Legumes and corn silage fiber digests and passes from the rumen quickly compared to perennial grasses and can be an excellent source of forage fiber for high producing cows. Fiber-turnover through the rumen is influenced by many factors, these includes intrinsic plant characteristics such as fiber content, particle size, fragility (rate of particle size reduction) and digestibility (rate of fermentation), and extrinsic factors within the rumen environment, such as rumination, absorption of fermentation end products, rumen pH and growth of the microbial population. The fiber fraction generally becomes more lignified, as forage matures, and the degree of fiber lignifications is directly related to the filling effects of the fiber within a forage type. Fiber that is less lignified are more digestible and clears from the rumen faster, allowing more space for the next meal. Selecting forages with high fiber digestibility can increase their feeding value. Alternatively, lignin degrading enzymes can also improve fiber digestibility, however the effect is not consistent. Some fungi specifically degrade lignin in cell walls, and can improve fiber digestibility in low quality fibrous materials such as crop residues. Improving the intake and digestion of fiber in dairy cows will result in a more efficient conversion of this non-digestible food resource into high-quality animal products. The total digestion of fiber is the major determinant of its energy value, however, rate of digestion and physical properties play an important role in maintaining rumen health.

Chapter 6 - Dietary fiber is a common and important ingredient in food product development. Its presence in food is desirable not only due to nutritional benefits but also for their functional and technological properties. In the present work, the rheology of four fiber fractions was evaluated. Two of them were obtained from quince waste which was submitted to different isolation processes: one with an ethanol treatment prior to drying and the other with distilled water washing previous to drying. The other fiber fractions were prepared from fresh peach pulp or peel. Suspensions of the fractions in deionized water were studied through dynamic tests. Weak gels of similar mechanical spectra were obtained when 2% w/w of peach fiber or 10% w/w of quince fiber suspensions were prepared in aqueous medium. Carbohydrate characteristics, particle size distribution and polidispersity influenced the rheological behavior. Mineral content was found to contribute to fiber nutritional value. Special attention should be paid to the process applied for the obtention of dietary fiber concentrates in order to assure their adequate functionality.

Chapter 7 - According to many scientific studies, people who have a diet rich in fiber have a low incidence of gastrointestinal disorders, diabetes mellitus, obesity and cardiovascular disease. An alternative to compensate the deficiency of dietary fiber in foods is to incorporate it as a supplement.

Pectin is a fermentable dietary fiber as it resists digestion and absorption in the human small intestine and experiences a total or partial fermentation in the large intestine. Besides possessing multiple health benefits, pectin has applications in the food industry as a gelling agent, thickener, fat replacement, emulsion stabilizer, among others.

In the industry, pectin is usually extracted by treating the raw material (i.e., apple, citrus) with dilute mineral acid at pH near 2, generating large amounts of effluents in need of treatment. Enzymatic methods of pectin isolation are an environmentally friendly alternative to acidic methods usually used and allow labeling products with ecological connotations tending to promote the consumption of products with these features. On the other hand, the increased consumption of fresh cut and peeled products generates a huge amount of wastes that is usually discarded; its use to obtain pectin can help to reduce pollution and restore biomass and nutrients.

The isolation techniques and characteristics of different fractions of dietary fiber isolated from industrialization wastes (leaves, stems, rhizomes and peels) of *Beta vulgaris* var. *conditiva* were studied in this research. The cell wall material was obtained through drying and grinding of *Beta vulgaris* wastes and its treatment with boiling ethanol rendered the alcohol insoluble residue. To isolate pectin enriched fractions, two different pre-treatments were assayed: one with sodium carbonate and another one with sodium hydroxide. The last one was selected because of the high yields and the product obtained was subjected to enzymatic digestion with cellulase and hemicellulase to obtain previously cited fractions. The highest antioxidant activity was detected in the cell wall material. The highest yield of the pectin enriched fractions was observed for the sodium hydroxide treatment followed by hydrolysis with cellulase. Rheological characterization showed pseudoplastic behavior with yield stress in flow assays. Dynamic assays showed weak gel behavior for all pectin enriched fractions in the presence of $CaCl_2$. Carbohydrate characteristics and polyphenol content influenced the antioxidant activity and rheological behavior.

Isolated fractions exhibited different technological characteristics and may be applied as food additives or ingredients.

Chapter 8 - *Objective:* Ovarian cancer is the third most common gynecological malignancy and the eighth leading cause of cancer-related deaths among women worldwide. The present study aimed to investigate the association between dietary fiber intake and the risk of epithelial ovarian cancer in southern Chinese women.

Methods: A case-control study was undertaken in Guangzhou, Guangdong Province, between 2006 and 2008. Participants were 500 incident ovarian cancer patients and 500 hospital-based controls. Information on habitual foods consumption was obtained by face-to-face interview, from which dietary fiber intakes were estimated using the Chinese food composition tables. Unconditional logistic regression analyses were performed to assess the association between dietary fiber intake and the ovarian cancer risk.

Results: The ovarian cancer patients reported lower intake levels of total dietary fiber and fiber derived from vegetables, fruits and cereals than those of controls. Overall, regular intake of fiber was inversely associated with the ovarian cancer risk, the adjusted odds ratio being 0.09 (95% confidence interval 0.05 to 0.14) for the highest (> 21.9 g) versus the lowest (< 16.5 g) tertile of daily intake, with a significant dose-response relationship ($p < 0.001$). Similar reduction in risk was also apparent for high intake level of vegetable fiber, but to a lesser extent for fruit fiber and cereal fiber.

Conclusion: Habitual intake of dietary fiber was inversely associated with the incidence of epithelial ovarian cancer in southern Chinese women.

Chapter 9 - Recently, the use of alternative fiber sources obtained from agroindustrial sub-products as fruit peels. Meat extenders comprise material that improve water retention (yield) and texture in cooked meat products. The most employed are potato starch and kappa carrageenan. The interaction of these three ingredients in a cooked sausage formulation was studied by means of a mixture design approach. Fiber in orange peel flour increased moisture and water retention, besides decreased oxidative rancidity in cooked sausages. Orange peel flour reduced sausages luminosity and redness, increasing yellowness. Fiber contained in orange peel flour improving texture resulting in softer but more cohesive and resilient sausages. Cooked meat products conditions (temperature and ionic strength) affected the functionality of meat extenders like potato starch and carrageenan. This indicates that orange peel flour as a cheap and viable fiber source can replace more expensive meat extenders, as potato starch or carrageenan.

Chapter 10 - Traditional polysaccharides obtained from plants may suffer from a lack of reproducibility in their rheological properties, purity, supply and cost. Most of the used plant polysaccharides are chemically modified to improve their characteristics. Microbial exopolysaccharides (EPSs) are principally composed of carbohydrate polymers, and they are produced by many microorganisms including bacteria, yeasts and fungi. Microorganisms can synthesize EPSs and excrete them out of cell either as soluble or insoluble polymers. These EPSs are able not only to protect the microorganisms themselves against desiccation, phage attack, antibiotics or toxic compounds, but also can be applied in several biotechnological applications. In food products they increase the dietary fiber content and can be used as viscosifiers, stabilizers, emulsifiers or gelling agents to improve physical and structural properties of water and oil holding capacity, viscosity, texture, sensory characteristics and shelf-life. EPSs are used as additives in various foods, such as dairy products, jams and jellies, wine and beer, fishery and meat products, icings and glazes, frozen foods and bakery products. Over the past few decades, interest in using microbial EPSs in food processing has been increasing because of main reasons such as easy production, better rheological and stability characteristics, cost effectiveness and supply. Dextran, xanthan, pullulan, curdlan, levan, gellan and alginate are the main examples of industrially important microbial exopolysaccharides. They also play crucial role in conferring beneficial physiological effects on human health, such as the ability to lower pressure and to reduce lipid level in blood. Furthermore, these EPSs exhibit antitumor, immunomodulating, antioxidant and antibacterial properties. The utility of various biopolymers are dependent on their monosaccharide composition, type of linkages present, degree of branching and molecular weight. In the present chapter, an attempt was taken to recapitulate the most important polysaccharides isolated from microorganisms as well as the main methods for microbial exopolysaccharide production, purification and structural characterization. In addition, the functional and healthy benefits of EPSs and their applications in food industry were discussed.

In: Dietary Fiber
Editor: Marvin E. Clemens
ISBN: 978-1-63463-655-1
© 2015 Nova Science Publishers, Inc.

Chapter 1

RESISTANT STARCH

Mindy Maziarz, Parakat Vijayagopal, Shanil Juma, Victorine Imrhan and Chandan Prasad
Department of Nutrition and Food Science,
Texas Woman's University, Denton, TX, US

ABSTRACT

Starch is a polysaccharide abundant in nature that undergoes hydrolysis in the small intestine to provide energy in the form of glucose.

Portions of starch resistant to hydrolysis that escape the small intestine and enter the large intestine intact to undergo fermentation is known as resistant starch (RS). Fivetypes of RS, 1-5, have been identified based on the physical inaccessibility, structure, retrogradation, or chemical modification of starch found either naturally or added to food. Thus, RS can be classified as a dietary or functional fiber. The formulation of ingredients containing RS by the food industry, such as high-amylose maize, can increase the fiber content of food without altering physiochemical or sensory attributes. The small molecular size, bland flavor, and white color, make RS an ideal partial replacement for fully-digestible starch in food.

A reduction in caloric availability is observed when RS replaces fully-digestible starch and can attenuate postprandial glucose and insulin concentrations. Additional physiological effects of RS result from the production of short chain fatty acids upon fermentation in the large intestine. RS improves digestive health by acting as a prebiotic, decreasing intestinal pH, and the formation of cancer-causing agents.

In murine models, dietary RS is associated with reductions in total and abdominal adiposity and improvements in lean mass. Increases in intestinal-derived satiety hormones, such as peptide YY and glucagon-like peptide-1, contribute to these findings. Despite mixed results associated with changes in blood glucose and insulin concentrations after long-term RS consumption, adults consuming 15-40 g daily have shown improvements in insulin sensitivity, particularly among those with metabolic syndrome.

RS is a functional fiber that can increase dietary fiber intake and positively impact overall health when consumed in adequate amounts.

INTRODUCTION

Over half of human energy needs are provided in the form of complex and simple carbohydrates. Complex carbohydrates include oligo- and poly-saccharides with three or more monomeric sugar units which provide approximately half of the total daily carbohydrate intake. Foods rich in complex carbohydrates include starchy vegetables, cereals, legumes, and whole grains. The other half of the dietary carbohydrate intake includes simple di- and mono-saccharides found in fruit, dairy, sugar-sweetened beverages and snacks, and many processed foods. Health professionals recommend lower intakes of simple carbohydrates, especially those added to foods, relative to complex carbohydrates. Simple carbohydrates are rapidly digested and absorbed in the small intestine and often provide limited nutritional value.

Starch is a glucose homopolysaccharide tightly packed into storage granules in plants. Two types of starch polymers exist and are classified according to the glycosidic linkage between specific carbons: amylose and amylopectin. Amylose has linear α-D-(1-4) bonds while amylopectin entails both branched α-D-(1-6) and linear α-D-(1-4) bonds (Leszczynski 2004). Starch typically contains 15-30% amylose but the percentage varies according to plant species (Sharma, Yadav, & Ritika, 2008). Additionally, plant breeding techniques can alter the amylose:amylopectin ratio. Higher amylose concentrations often correlate with decreased digestibility because of its linear molecular structure (Birt et al., 2013).

This review focuses on the classification, dietary sources, and health benefits of a type of starch that resists digestion in the small intestine classified as resistant starch (RS). The majority of research examining the impact of RS on health include RS Type 2 (RS2) instead of other types of RS; therefore, this review focuses mostly on the studies examining RS2 intake.

Classification of RS

In the small intestine, α-amylase and α-dextrinase act upon α-D-(1-4) and α-D-(1-6) glycosidic bonds of starch respectively, to form glucose. However, the hydrolysis of starch in the small intestine can vary based on granular structure, physical properties, retrogradation, and/or chemical modification (Sharma, Yadav, & Ritika, 2008). Englyst, Kingman, and Cummings (1992) identified three categories of starch based on the rate and amount hydrolyzed in the small intestine: rapidly digested, slowly digested, and resistant to digestion. Rapidly digestible starch undergoes fast, complete digestion, while slowly digestible starch is fully hydrolyzed within 120 minutes following enzymatic action by pancreatic amylase and glucosidase. The portion of starch not digested in the small intestine, thus entering the large intestine intact is known as RS. There are five types of RS (RS1 to RS5) that can occur naturally in foods, form during processing, or result from chemical or physical modification. RS1 is physically inaccessible to digestive enzymes therefore resists hydrolysis. The crystalline-type granular structure of RS2 is prevalent in starchy foods, like potatoes and just-ripe bananas, do not undergo enzymatic cleavage. However, cooking RS2 can alter its granular structure and improve digestibility. High-amylose maize, a type of RS2 resulting from a genetic alteration in corn that contains high amylose concentrations, maintains resistance to digestibility even at high temperatures. Retrogradation is the process of cooking then cooling starches that forms RS3. This process makes RS3 quite heat-stable, which is often ideal for food processing. RS4 is produced by chemical-modification such as esterification or cross-linking that inhibits enzymatic digestion. A fifth type of RS, resistant maltodextrins, is also heat-stable and produced from the interaction of lipids or other molecules that form aggregates (Frohberg & Quanz, 2008) or from the rearrangement of the starch molecules to maintain resistance (Mermelstein, 2009). The classification of RS and respective food sources are listed in Table 1.

Table 1. Classification of Resistant Starch (RS)*

Type of RS	Starch Properties	Food Sources
Type 1	Physically inaccessible	Partially milled grains, seeds, and kernals
Type 2	Resistant granules	Raw potato; just-ripe bananas; high-amylose maize; legumes
Type 3	Retrograded	Cooked then cooled foods, such as potatoes, cereals, breads, and corn flakes; foods undergoing moist/heat treatment
Type 4	Chemically- or physically-modified starches to form new resistant bonds, such as cross-links, esters or ethers.	Foods enriched or enhanced with fiber
Type 5	Resistant maltodextrins	Foods with starch and lipid

*Sources: Englyst et al., 1992; Haub et al., 2010; Homayouni et al., 2014; Nugent 2005.

RS can be either a dietary (endogenous to food) or functional (added to food) fiber. While RS1 and RS2 are dietary fibers, RS3 and RS4 are considered functional fibers. According to the Dietary Reference Intakes: Proposed Definition of Dietary Fiber (2001) report, dietary fiber is described as "nondigestible carbohydrates and lignin that are intrinsic and intact in plants," (p. 22), while functional fibers are those carbohydrates that are isolated and provide a physiological benefit due to their non-digestible nature (Institute of Medicine, Food and Nutrition Board, 2001). Total fiber is the sum of dietary and functional fibers. A more recent definition established by the Codex Alimentarius Commission describes dietary fiber as carbohydrate polymers with $\geq$ 10 monomeric units that resist small intestine enzyme hydrolysis (Codex Alimentarius, 2008). The polymeric carbohydrates can be broken down into three categories: those that are edible and naturally occurring in food; those obtained from raw food by physical, enzymatic, or chemical means to provide physiological health benefits; and those that are synthetic and have scientifically proven physiological benefits.

Dietary Intake and Food Sources

Average global intakes of RS are between 3 and 10 g/day (Glodring 2004). In the Chinese population, the daily RS consumption is reported at 14.9 g, which is currently above the global average (Chen et al., 2010). High-RS food sources in this population include tubers and cereals. According to a National Nutrition Survey, Australians consume between 3.4 and 9.4 g RS daily (Roberts et al., 2004). The average RS intake in Europe from 1993-94 was 4.1 g/d (Dysseler & Hoffem, 1994), while the United States (U.S.) averaged 4.9 g/d (range 2.8-7.9 g/d), based on data from the 1999-2002 National Health and Human Nutrition Examination survey (Murphy, Douglass, & Birkett, 2008). In the U.S., bread, cooked cereals and pasta, vegetables, bananas/plantains, and legumes were the top five sources of dietary RS (Murphy et al., 2008). Other processed foods, such as cakes, chips, breakfast cereals, and cookies/crackers also contribute to the total daily RS intake. Table 2 represents foods with ≥3.0 g RS per 100 g of food, according to a database of RS-containing foods created by Murphy et al., 2008. The amount of RS inherently found in the same food type, however, can vary according to growing location and conditions, ripeness, and cooking method.

Table 2. Foods with ≥3.0 g RS per 100 g

Food Type	g of RS per 100 g Food
Oats, rolled, raw	11.3
Puffed wheat	6.2
Pumpernickel bread	4.5
Beans, white, cooked and/or canned	4.2
Rice square cereal	4.2
Banana, raw	4.0
Italian bread, toasted	3.8
Rye bread, wholemeal	3.2
Chips, potato	3.5
Plantain, cooked	3.5
Lentils	3.4
Mucsli	3.3

Source: Murphy et al., 2008.

RS Properties As a Food Ingredient

RS is an ideal food ingredient because of its physical properties and unique characteristics. RS is white, bland, and odorless, and composed of small-sized granules (1.2 x 10^5 Da) with low water holding capacity (Sajilata, Singhal, & Kulkarni, 2006; Tharanathan, 2002). Although many foods inherently contain RS, food manufacturing companies have formulated high RS ingredients utilizing a variety of methods: hydrolysis by an enzyme or acid, hydrothermal treatments, retrogradation, or cross-linking (Ozturk & Koksel, 2014). One example of a natural high-RS ingredient is Hi-Maize® 260 corn starch that contains approximately 60% RS2 and 40% fully digestible starch. Hi-Maize® 260 is a desirable ingredient because its intrinsic properties are maintained during food processing and preparation and is gluten-free (Nugent 2005). Other high-RS commercial ingredients include Hylon VII (RS2), Novelose 240 (RS2), Novelose 330 (RS3) and Fibersym® RW (RS4).

The high-RS ingredients are often incorporated into foods as a way to improve the nutritional profile of the food while maintaining overall consumer acceptability. For example, as much as 20% of digestible starch can be replaced with high RS ingredients in gluten-free bread products without compromising organoleptic properties (Korus et al., 2009). We found that partially-replacing fully-digestible flour with RS2 in medium-sized muffins (113 g) to provide 3.21 g RS2 does not impact the over likeability when compared to control (Maziarz et al., 2012). RS can also be added to pasta products while maintaining texture, color, and quality, especially when compared to other types of fiber-enriched pastas (Homayouni et al., 2014). Aside from baked goods, the incorporation of high RS2 ingredients in fried foods can maintain consumer acceptability (Sanz, Salvador, & Fiszman, 2008). RS2 and RS3 incorporated into cheese can lower fat content (Noronha, O'Riordan, & O'Sullivan, 2007) and up to 18% or RS2 can be added to cheese without impacting texture or overall acceptability (Duggan et al., 2008). Use of flour blends high in RS can partially or completely replace the fully-digestible flour in baked goods or casseroles or can be incorporated into smoothies, cereals, and yogurt.

Quantification of RS

The Codex Alimentarius approves several methods for analyzing total dietary fiber, including Association of Official Analytical Chemists (AOAC) 991.43, 985.29, and 2009.01, but these methods may not measure total RS concentrations due to differences in solubility and thermostability between RS types (McCleary et al., 2013). The AOAC 2002.02 is the approved method for determining RS. Depending on the type of RS in the food sample, the AOAC 991.43 method, which includes a boiling step and treatment with an enzyme, may be adequate. However, more specific RS quantification methods may be more suitable for other types of RS, especially for those that are non-heat stable. For example, comparing the RS method AOAC 2002.02 with the dietary fiber method AOAC 991.43 produced similar results for two commercial RS products: Nuvelose 204 and Nuvelose 330 (McCleary et al., 2013). In contrast, a large portion of RS was not captured with the AOAC 991.43 method for the native potato starch, Actistar, and green banana because the RS in these foods become soluble when heated. However, the AOAC 2002.02 method adequately captured the RS in these foods (McCleary et al., 2013).

The duration of enzymatic treatment may also impact RS determination. The Englyst method indirectly measures RS and employs a 2 hour enzymatic incubation period in contrast to the 16 hour incubation period of AOAC 2002.02 that measures RS directly (Englyst et al., 2013). Englyst et al. (2013) concluded that AOAC 2002.02 more accurately quantified RS3 versus RS2 due to the lower enzyme concentration and increased incubation period that allowed for adequate hydrolysis of the starch granule. The RS2 in raw flours were more accurately analyzed using the Englyst starch method instead of the AOAC 2002.02 method (Englyst et al., 2013).

Furthermore, adequate RS4 analysis transpires between 40-60°C because temperatures above 100°C promote gelatinization of the starch granule and decrease enzymatic hydrolysis (McCleary et al., 2013). Quantifying RS4 using method employing very high temperatures would overestimate the amount of RS4 available to humans at physiological conditions.

In summary, accurate quantification of RS content in foods depends on the type of RS being analyzed and utilization of the appropriate method.

RS Impact on Digestive Health

The fermentation of RS by microorganisms in the large intestine contributes to digestive health. In addition to methane and hydrogen gas, short-chain fatty acids (SCFA) are the most physiologically relevant products of fermentation. Acetate and propionate, two of the SCFAs absorbed and utilized by the muscle and liver, respectively, provide up to 10-15% of daily energy requirements. Another SCFA, butyrate provides energy to large intestine epithelial cells and assists in cell proliferation, gene expression, and maintaining the integrity of the mucosal wall (Brownawell et al., 2012). RS promotes digestive health by enhancing mineral absorption secondary to reductions in pH, improves laxation, and decreases diarrheal incidence and duration (Brownawell et al., 2012; Murphy et al., 2008; Topping & Clifton, 2001). In addition, RS is classified as a prebiotic and improves the growth of beneficial bacterial, such as *bifidobacteria* and *lactobacilli*, in the colon to provide health benefits to the host (I. Brown, Wang, Topping, Playne, & Conway, 1998; Roberfroid et al., 2010). The insoluble properties of RS do not contribute to fecal bulk like viscous fibers; however, the increased bacterial load can contribute to bulking and mass.

RS is well tolerated in most individuals, especially when compared to similar intake amounts of other functional fibers. For example, fructooligosaccharides and inulin are fructose polymers that are rapidly fermented in the large intestine and can produce undesirable gastrointestinal (GI) side effects, such as gas, bloating, and abdominal pain when ≥ 15 g/d are consumed (Maziarz 2013). Consuming approximately twice the amount of RS2 (30 g) as fructose polymers is adequately tolerated in most individuals (Grabitske & Slavin, 2009). The following factors can impact the GI tolerance of RS: type, duration of intake, amount consumed at one sitting, and the presence of additional nutrients if RS is consumed as mixed-meal (Grabitske & Slavin, 2009). Studies examining the consumption of 30 – 40 g RS2 daily over a period of 4-12 weeks show GI tolerability with only minor symptoms reported. One study by Maki et al. (2012) examined the intake of 30 g RS2 daily in overweight adults for 4 weeks. One-third of the participants reported increased flatulence in this study, but the severity of GI symptoms did not impact degree of compliance to the dietary protocol (Maki et al., 2012). Other studies of longer duration (8 and 12 weeks) found that overweight adults also adequately tolerated the daily consumption of 40 g RS2 (Johnston, Thomas, Bell, Frost, & Robertson, 2010; Robertson et al., 2012). In contrast, ingesting larger amounts of RS2 (~60 g) over a period of 24 hours produced undesirable GI effects, such as mild diarrhea, increased flatulence, and more frequent defecation in healthy adults (Muir et al., 1995).

Energy Contribution of RS

Isolated RS does not directly contribute to energy requirements, but rather indirectly through the peripheral metabolism of absorbed acetate and propionate resulting from microbiota fermentation in the large intestine. Over 90% of SCFA can be absorbed across the epithelial lining of the large intestine, thus the consumption of RS in large quantities (≥20 g) can contribute substantial amounts of energy, albeit less than the average 4.2 kcal/g obtained from fully-digestible carbohydrates (Behall and Howe, 1995; Wong et al., 2006; Sharma 2008). A high-amylose diet (70%) was estimated to provide only 63% of the energy contribution of cornstarch; however, the digestion of RS can have intra-individual variation (Behall and Howe, 1996). Behall and Howe (1996) found that healthy adults who were age- and weight-matched with hyperinsulinemic adults digested 81.8% of the RS to provide 3.4 kcal/g. The hyperinsulinemic adults digested only 53.2% and received 2.2 kcal/g from the RS (Behall & Howe, 1996). The discrepancies in digestive properties of RS observed could be related to the microbiota profile and presence of other dietary compounds in the large intestine. For example, non-starch polysaccharide excretion in the feces can increase by 50% with the consumption of a high-RS diet (39 g/d), although the impact on total caloric intake and body weight did not differ from the low-RS diet (5 g/d) (Phillips et al., 1995). The partial replacement of RS with fully digestible starch can lower the caloric value of food, but the energy contribution from SCFA must also be considered. Likewise, commercial ingredients used in many animal and human studies, such as Hi-Maize 260®, contain approximately 60% RS while the remaining 40% digestible starch will contribute to energy requirments.

Subjective Satiety and RS

Promoting satiety is one proposed mechanism by which RS may reduce body weight and lower obesity incidence. Subjective satiety, or the perceived fullness after consuming food, is often measured by either a visual analogue scale (VAS) or 7-point bipolar scale. Studies examining the impact of RS on satiety and fullness show mixed results. Using a 7-point bipolar scale (-3 extra hungry, 0 neutral, +3 fully satiated), healthy adults were more satiated after consuming approximately 30 g RS2 and RS3 for 10 days (Jenkins et al.,1998). Another study utilized a VAS to measure satiety in healthy adults consuming isocaloric muffins with different types of fiber. The RS2 muffins (8 g RS2) produced a high satiation score up to three hours postprandially (Willis et al., 2009). In contrast, two studies found no change in satiety after RS consumption. One study found no change in subjective satiety measured by a VAS after adults consumed 27.2 g RS or 27.2 RS plus pullulan at breakfast when compared to a low-fiber control (Klosterbuer, Thomas, & Slavin, 2012). Another study did not find differences in satiety measured by a VAS, but a significant reduction in energy at a subsequent *ad libitum* meal and over 24 hours after consuming 48 g RS2 equally divided between breakfast and lunch (Bodinham et al., 2010). We found a 24.2% improvement in overall mean subjective satiety score measured by a VAS after overweight adults consumed 30 g RS2 in muffins for 6 weeks (n = 13) compared to a 0.59% overall mean change in the placebo (n = 7) (Maziarz et al., 2014, unpublished data). However, statistical significance was not achieved likely due to small sample size. We also did not observe a reduction in body weight in the RS2 group despite the change in subjective satiety.

The Influence of RS on Gut-derived Satiety Hormones and Adiposity

Appetite and energy expenditure are regulated synergistically by neuronal and hormonal signals between the GI tract and central nervous system (Geraedts, Troost, & Saris, 2011; Cummings & Overduin, 2007). Satiety is one factor associated with appetite and is defined as the length of time between the cessation of one meal and the beginning of the next meal. Thus improving satiety would decrease appetite. The presence of food in the GI tract promotes gastric distention to stimulate vagus afferents that converge at the hindbrain and provide feedback responses that control digestion, GI motility, and satiety (Ritter, 2004; Cummings & Overduin, 2007; Dockray, 2013). The direct presence of food in the GI tract and the physical and chemical properties of the food elicit the release of gut-derived hormones, such as peptide tyrosine tyrosine (PYY) and glucagon-like peptide-1 (GLP-1), which can also travel to the hindbrain and arcuate nucleus to influence satiety and energy expenditure (Ritter, 2004; Cummings & Overduin 2007). In addition to impacting the satiety center of the brain, additional mechanisms can contribute to gut-derived hormonal satiation. GLP-1 is a well-known incretin that upregulates glucose-mediated insulin release (Murphy & Bloom, 2006; Holst, 2007). Synergistically, GLP-1 and PYY inhibit GI tract motility and emptying by stimulating the "ileal brake" that can further promote a sensation of fullness (Maljaars et al., 2008). The hormones also demonstrate a more pronounced impact on satiety by reducing caloric intake by 27%, which was sustained over a 24 hour period, when co-administered intravenously than when administered individually (Neary et al., 2005).

The SCFA produced from RS fermentation can promote the release of PYY and GLP-1 from the L-enteroendocrine cells by binding to the free fatty acid transmembrane receptors (FFAR) 2 and 3, also known as G protein-coupled receptors 43 and 41, respectively (Xiong et al., 2004; Lin et al., 2012). Acetate preferentially binds to FFAR2, butyrate binds to FFAR3, while propionate binds to both receptors (Brown et al., 2003; Lin et al., 2012). The addition of SCFA simulating the concentrations of the human large intestine (acetate (80 mmol/L), propionate (40 mmol/L), and butyrate (20 mmol/L)) to murine colonic cells increased GLP-1 release by 1.3 fold (Tolhurst et al., 2012). A 70% reduction in GLP-1 production was observed with propionate incubation of FFAR2 knockout mice cell cultures, while acetate completely eliminated GLP-1 release (Tolhurst et al., 2012). Likewise, another study found a significant increase in GLP-1 after the oral administration of propionate and butyrate in mice; however, FFAR3 knockout mice showed a blunted GLP-1 response after butyrate, but not propionate, administration (Lin et al., 2012). The impact of SCFAs on FFAR2 and FFAR3 expression in the large intestine in humans after RS consumption remains to be explored.

In many animal models, RS2 demonstrates a notable impact on gut-derived satiety hormones and adiposity. The administration of a RS2-rich (approximately 30% wt/wt) diet decreased overall and abdominal adiposity when compared to control even when energy contributions of the diets remain similar (Keenan et al., 2006; Shen et al., 2008; Keenan et al., 2013). Increased GLP-1 and PYY concentrations (Keenan et al., 2006; Shen et al., 2008; Zhou et al. 2008), as well as proglucagon and PYY gene expression (Keenan et al., 2006; Zhou et al., 2008) contribute to these findings. One study found that obese mice did not ferment RS due to the lack of pH change in the large intestine and no reduction in body fat was observed when compared to C57BL/6J mice (Zhou et al., 2009). In contrast, Keenen et al. (2013) found that ovariectomized rats consuming RS2 increased bacteria concentrations and subsequent fermentation of RS in the large intestine, and a reduction in abdominal fat resulted. Collectively, these studies suggest fermentation of RS in the large intestine plays a physiological role in reducing body fat in animal models. Interestingly, another rat study found decreased body fat with increased PYY and GLP-1concentrations after RS2 intake, but a reduction in food intake was not observed (Shen et al., 2008). The upregulation of energy expenditure by proopiomelanocortin neuron stimulation measured by gene expression may have contributed to the decrease in body fat (Shen et al., 2008).

To date, human trials examining RS2 consumption have not resulted in favorable changes in gut-derived satiety hormones, adiposity, or overall body weight. One study found that despite a near significant increase in propionate, GLP-1 concentrations did not differ the morning after healthy individuals consumed either 60 g RS2 or placebo divided into four portions throughout the day (Robertson et al., 2003). Another study examined the incremental area under the curve (iAUC) for GLP-1 in healthy males after the ingestion of 48 g RS2 equally divided between a breakfast and lunch meal (Bodingham et al., 2013). Compared to the control meals of similar energy and digestible carbohydrate content, the iAUC GLP-1 significantly decreased after the RS2 breakfast meal with no change after the lunch meal. Another study found a decrease in iAUC GLP-1 after adults consumed 27.2 g RS + pullulan at breakfast (Klosterbuer, Thomas, & Slavin, 2012). The duration of these studies may be too short to depict changes in gut-derived satiety hormones associated with RS fermentation.

Studies of longer duration (≥4 weeks) also have not found a relationship between gut-derived satiety hormones and adiposity. The consumption of 30 g RS2/d in healthy adults over four weeks did not change body weight, adiposity, or GLP-1 concentrations; however, a small, but significant increase in lean body mass resulted (Robertson et al., 2005). Another study examined the impact of consuming 67 g RS2/d for eight weeks in adults with metabolic syndrome and reported no change in body weight, adiposity, or lean body mass (Robertson et al., 2012). Two other studies examining the influence of 15 g and 30 g RS2/d for four weeks and 40 g RS2/d for 12 weeks in individuals with metabolic syndrome also found no change in body weight or adiposity (Johnston et al., 2010; Maki et al., 2012). Bodingham et al. (2014) found increases in fasting propionate and butyrate but decrease in fasting GLP-1 after individuals with Type 2 Diabetes Mellitus (T2DM) consumed 40 g RS2 daily for 12 weeks; however, the postprandial iAUC GLP-1 was higher after a meal tolerance test. No changes in body weight, BMI, or fat mass were observed in this study.

Interestingly, while changes in body weight or adiposity have not been reported after RS2 interventions, alterations in adipose tissue modeling have occurred. Adipose tissue modeling can provide insight into the physiological changes observed after RS2 intake, such as improvements in insulin sensitivity (S_I). One study examining the acute ingestion of a 5.7% HAM-RS2 breakfast meal found increased fat oxidation when compared to an isocaloric control meal with equal amounts of fat and fiber, although differences in digestible carbohydrates could have contributed to the findings (Higgins et al., 2004). As reported above, Robertson et al. (2012) found a two-fold increase in adipose hormone-sensitive lipase and lipoprotein lipase gene expression, as well as the expression of other genes involved in fat metabolism among individuals with metabolic syndrome after consuming 40 g RS2 daily for 8 weeks. A lower insulin-stimulated non-esterified fatty acid (NEFA) release was also found after RS2 intake, which could be explained by peripheral SCFA actions on adipocytes (Robertson et al., 2012). However, despite an increase in adiponectin gene expression in adipocytes, changes in fasting plasma adiponectin concentrations did not transpire (Robertson et al., 2012). Likewise, fasting leptin concentrations also did not change in this study. We found a significant decrease in iAUC leptin in overweight adults (n = 13) after the consumption of 30 g RS2 daily from muffins for six weeks (Maziarz et al., 2014 unpublished data). Interestingly, these results occurred despite no change in overall fat mass suggesting the possibility of adipocyte modeling. Leptin is an adipokine that circulates in the blood proportionally to fat mass and larger adipocytes release more leptin (Skurk et al., 2007). Additional research is needed to determine the mechanistic actions associated with SCFA and adipocyte lipolysis or remodeling. Table 3 compares fatty acid metabolism after RS2 consumption in studies of longer duration.

Robertson (2005) reviewed several factors that contribute to the lack of translatability from animals to human studies when examining the impact of gut-derived satiety hormones on adiposity with RS intake. First, the animals ingest very high amounts of RS, up to 30-50% total dietary weight, which is physiologically impossible for humans. Second, animals have a greater large intestine to total body weight ratio than humans; therefore, animals have the ability to produce more fecal mass. The microbiota profile, which impacts the fermentation of RS, may also differ between species. Lastly, humans receive RS after the establishment of adipose tissue has been established, while animals often receive the RS intervention before adipose tissue deposition begins.

RS, Blood Glucose, and Insulin Resistance

RS2 is not hydrolyzed by small intestine enzymes; therefore, the direct contribution of RS to blood glucose concentrations are null. The partial or full replacement of fully-digestible starch in a food product with RS2 (or a high-RS2 flour) would lower the amount of glucose available to the blood and lower postprandial glucose concentrations. Thus, studies examining the impact of RS2 on blood glucose and insulin concentrations should have equal amounts of fully-digestible starch so the true impact of RS2 on the metabolic profile can be determined. Studies examining the intake of RS while controlling the amount of fully-digestible starch are presented below and in Table 3.

The type of RS consumed can impact glucose response. In healthy adults, drinking 30 g RS4 in water elicited a significantly lower iAUC glucose postprandial response over 120 minutes than 30 g RS2 (Haub et al., 2010). Interestingly, the RS4 had 91.9% dietary fiber, while the RS2 had 83% fiber. In contrast, a study of longer duration (12 weeks) found no significant change in fasting or postprandial glucose after adults consumed RS4 enriched flour (30% v/v) incorporated into a variety of foods (Nichenametla et al., 2013).

The short-term impact of RS2 on blood glucose and insulin show mixed results and may be related to the amount of RS2 administered. Robertson et al. (2003) administered 60 g RS2 to healthy adults throughout the day, then administered a meal tolerance test the following morning. Postprandial blood glucose and insulin, as well as increased insulin sensitivity ($S_{I\ (oral)}$) occurred. Another study found a decrease in postprandial insulin without changes in blood glucose in healthy males receiving 48 g RS2 divided over two meals, and measurements of insulin sensitivity did not change (Bodingham, Frost, and Robertson, 2010).

Studies of longer duration suggest that RS2 exhibits a more pronounced impact on peripheral S_I than blood glucose or insulin concentrations. In healthy adults, peripheral S_I improved alongside suppressed adipose tissue lipolysis after the consumption of 30 g RS2 daily for four weeks (Robertson et al., 2005).

Three studies examining RS2 intake among adults with metabolic syndrome or insulin resistance also found improvements in peripheral S_I without notable changes in hepatic glucose output (Johnston et al., 2010; Maki et al., 2012; Robertson et al., 2012). The changes in S_I could be related to alterations in the NEFA release from adipocytes as prolonged plasma fatty acid concentrations impair pancreatic β-cell function and peripheral glucose uptake (Kashyap et al., 2003).

Table 3. Comparison of RS2 Intake, Blood Glucose, and Insulin Sensitivity in Long-term (≥4 weeks) Studies

Author/Year	Participants	Intervention/ Study Design	Method of Analysis	Plasma [Glucose] after RS2 Intake	Plasma [Insulin] after RS2 Intake	Insulin Sensitivity (S_I) after RS2 Intake	Fatty Acid Changes after RS2 Intake
Robertson et al., 2005	Healthy adults (n = 10)	30 g RS2 or placebo daily for 4 weeks, crossover	Euglycemic clamp; meal tolerance test	No change in fasting or iAUC	No change in fasting, iAUC decreased (*P*=0.024)	Increased in muscle (*P*=0.013) and adipose (*P*=0.007)	Decreased release from adipose (*P*=0.019), no change in muscle uptake
Johnston et al., 2010	Metabolic syndrome (n = 20)	40 g RS2 or placebo daily for 12 weeks, parallel	Euglycemic clamp; homeostasis model	Not reported	Not reported	Increased (19%) in peripheral (*P*=0.023); no change in HOMA %B or %S	No change
Robertson et al., 2012	Metabolic syndrome (n = 16)	40 g RS2 or placebo daily for 8 weeks, crossover	Euglycemic clamp; meal tolerance test; adipose biopsies	Decrease in fasting (*P*=0.029)	Decrease in fasting (*P*=0.041)	Decrease HOMA-IR by 10.4% (*P*=0.029); Increase peripheral Si by 21.1% after clamp; Increase forearm Si by 65% after MTT	Increase insulin suppression of NEFA (*P*=0.041) but 16% increase in fatty acid uptake in skeletal muscle during MTT (*P*=0.055)
Maki et al., 2012	Insulin Resistant (n = 33)	30 g RS2, 15 g RS2, or placebo daily for 4 weeks; crossover	Glucose tolerance test, homeostasis model	No change in fasting	No change in fasting	S_I increased in men after 15 g RS2 by 56.5% (*P*=0.031) and 30 g RS2 by 78.2% (*P*=0.019); no change in HOMA%S or HOMA%B	No change in total FFA
Bodinham et al., 2014	T2DM (n = 17)	40 g RS2 or placebo daily for 12 weeks, crossover	Euglycemic clamp; meal tolerance test	No change in fasting or $HbA1_c$; Decrease in postprandial iAUC glucose (*P*=0.036)	No change in fasting or postprandial	No change in HOMA%S or HOMA%B	Decrease in fasting NEFA (*P*=0.004); increase in insulin suppression of NEFA after clamp (*P*=0.001)

Note. iAUC = incremental area under the curve; HOMA = Homeostatic Model Assessment; MTT = meal tolerance test; NEFA = non-esterified fatty acids; S_I = insulin sensitivity; T2DM = Type 2 Diabetes Mellitus; $HbA1_c$ = hemoglobin A1.

Interestingly, improvements in S_I occurred despite the lack of change in ectopic fat stores in the soleus and tibialis (Johnston et al., 2010), or decreased fat stores in muscle even with increased fatty acid uptake (Robertson et al., 2012). The ectopic fat stores in muscle is one contributing factor implicated in the pathogenesis of insulin resistance (Guilherme et al., 2008). Despite improvements observed in S_I among adults with metabolic syndrome, 40 g RS2 daily for 12 weeks does not appear to impact S_I in adults with well-controlled T2DM. Bodinham et al. (2014) observed a decrease in fasting glucose and NEFA with improved insulin suppression of NEFA, but no change in either hepatic or peripheral S_I. In fact, soleus intramyocellular lipid depots increased. A significant 60-120 minute postprandial increase in GLP-1 was also observed in this study, despite a significant decrease in fasting GLP-1, which could partially explain the relationship between RS2 and lower postprandial iAUC glucose after the meal tolerance test (Bodinham et al., 2014).

Despite a few studies showing improvements in blood glucose and insulin concentrations following RS intake, the research suggests RS can improve S_I. The mechanism has not been fully elucidated, but the interrelationship between RS fermentation in the large intestine, peripheral SCFA concentrations, and changes in adipocyte modeling appear to play a role.

CONCLUSION

RS is an insoluble, fermentable fiber that can be added to many types of foods without impacting overall physiochemical properties or consumer acceptability while improving nutrient composition. The physiological benefits of RS, mostly related to the fermentation of RS, result from consuming adequate amounts over time. The caveat entails obtaining adequate amounts of RS ($\geq$15 g/day) from natural food sources instead of foods enhanced with high-RS2 ingredients to achieve the scientifically observed health-related benefits. The improvements in S_I shown after RS2 consumption appear to be more pronounced in individuals with insulin resistance or metabolic syndrome. However, all individuals, regardless of metabolic profile, can incorporate high-RS foods into their diet as a way to achieve daily dietary fiber goals.

REFERENCES

Behall, K. M., & Howe, J. C. (1995). Contribution of fiber and resistant starch to metabolizable energy. *The American Journal of Clinical Nutrition, 62*(5), 1158S-1160S.

Behall, K., & Howe, J. (1996). Resistant starch as energy. *Journal of the American College of Nutrition, 15*(3), 248-254.

Birt, D.F., Boylston, T., Hendrich, S., Jane, J-L., Hollis, J., Li, L., McClelland, J., Moore, S., Phillips, G.J., Rowling, M., Schalinske, K., Scott, M.P., Whitley, E.M. (2013). Resistant starch: Promise for improving human health. *Advances in Nutrition, 4*, 587-601.

Bodinham, C. L., Smith, L., Thomas, E. L., Bell, J. D., Swann, J. R., Costabile, A., Russell-Jones, D., Umpleby, A. M., Robertson, M. D. (2014). Efficacy of increased resistant starch consumption in human type 2 diabetes. *Endocrine Connections, 3*, 75-84.

Bodinham, C. L., Al-Mana, N. M., Smith, L., & Robertson, M. D. (2013). Endogenous plasma glucagon-like peptide-1 following acute dietary fibre consumption. *The British Journal of Nutrition, 110*(8), 1429-1433. doi:10.1017/S0007114513000731.

Bodinham, C. L., Frost, G. S., & Robertson, M. D. (2010). Acute ingestion of resistant starch reduces food intake in healthy adults. *The British Journal of Nutrition, 103*(6), 917-922.

Brown, I., Wang, X., Topping, D., Playne, M., & Conway, P. (1998). High amylose maize starch as a versatile prebiotic for use with probiotic bacteria. *Food Australia, 50*(12), 603-613.

Brownawell, A. M., Caers, W., Gibson, G. R., Kendall, C. W., Lewis, K. D., Ringel, Y., & Slavin, J. L. (2012). Prebiotics and the health benefits of fiber: Current regulatory status, future research, and goals. *The Journal of Nutrition, 142*(5), 962-974.

Chen, L., Liu, R., Qin, C., Meng, Y., Zhang, J., Wang, Y., Xu, G. (2010). Sources and intake of resistant starch in the Chinese diet. *Asia Pacific Journal of Clinical Nutrition, 19*(2), 274-282.

Codex Alimentarius. (2008). *Report of the 30th session of the codex committee on nutrition and foods for special dietary uses.* (No. ALINORM 09/32/26). Cape Town, South Africa.

Cummings, D. E., & Overduin, J. (2007). Gastrointestinal regulation of food intake. *Journal of Clinical Investigation, 117*(1), 13-23.

Dockray, G. J. (2013). Enteroendocrine cell signaling via the vagus nerve. *Current Opinion in Pharmacology, 13*(6), 954-958.

Duggan, E. Noronha, N., O'Riordan, E.D., O'Sullivan, M. (2008). Effect of resistant starch on the water binding properties of imitation cheese. *Journal Food Engineering, 84,* 108-115.

Dysseler, P. and Hoffem, D. (1994). Comparison between Englyst's method and Berry's modified method on 20 different starch foods. *Proceedings of the Concluding Plenary Meeting of EURESTA*. European FLAIR-Concerted Action: No. 11. (pp. 84-86).

Englyst, H. N., Kingman, S., & Cummings, J. (1992). Classification and measurement of nutritionally important starch fractions. *European Journal of Clinical Nutrition, 46*(2), S33-S50.

Englyst, K., Quigley, M., Englyst, H., Parmar, B., Damant, A., Elahi, S., Lawrence, P. (2013). Evaluation of methods of analysis for dietary fibre using real foods and model foods. *Food Chemistry, 14,* 568-573.

Frohberg, C., Quanz, M. (2008). Use of linear poly-alpha-1,4-glucans as resistant starch. *United States Patent Application No. 0249297 A1* United States of America, pp. 1-8.

Geraedts, M. C. P., Troost, F., & Saris, W. (2011). Gastrointestinal targets to modulate satiety and food intake. *Obesity Reviews, 12*(6), 470-477.

Goldring, J.M. (2004). Resistant Starch: Safe intakes and legal status. *Journal of AOAC, 87*(3), 733-739.

Grabitske, H.A., Slavin, J.L. (2009). Gastrointestinal effects of low-digestible carbohydrates. *Critical Reviews of Food Science and Nutrition, 49*, 327-360.

Guilherme, A., Virbasius, J.V., Puri, V., Czech, M.P. (2008). Adipocyte dysfunctions linking obesity to insulin resistance and type 2 diabetes. *Nature Reviews Molecular Cell Biology, 9*, 367-377.

Haub, M.D., Hubach, K.L., Al-tamimi, E.K., Ornelas, S., & Seib P.A. (2010). Different types of resistant starch elicit different glucose responses in humans. *Journal of Nutrition and Metabolism.* doi:10.1155/2010/230501

Higgins, J. A., Higbee, D. R., Donahoo, W. T., Brown, I. L., Bell, M. L., & Bessesen, D. H. (2004). Resistant starch consumption promotes lipid oxidation. *Nutrition & Metabolism, 1*(8.) doi:10.1186/1743-7075-1-8

Holst, J. J. (2007). The physiology of glucagon-like peptide 1. *Physiological Reviews, 87*(4), 1409-1439.

Homayouni, A., Amini, A., Keshtiban, A.K., Mortazavian, A.M., Esazadeh, K., Pourmoradian, S. (2014). Resistant starch in the food industry: A changing outlook for consumer and producer. *Starch, 66*, 102-114.

Institute of Medicine. Food and Nutrition Board. (2001). *Dietary reference intakes: Proposed definition of dietary fiber*. Washington, D.C.: The National Academies Press.

Jenkins, D. J., Vuksan, V., Kendall, C. W., Wursch, P., Jeffcoat, R., Waring, S, Mehling, C.C., Augustin, L.S., Wong, E. (1998). Physiological effects of resistant starches on fecal bulk, short chain fatty acids, blood lipids and glycemic index. *Journal of the American College of Nutrition, 17*(6), 609-616.

Johnston, K., Thomas, E., Bell, J., Frost, G., & Robertson, M. (2010). Resistant starch improves insulin sensitivity in metabolic syndrome. *Diabetic Medicine, 27*(4), 391-397.

Kashyap, S., Belfor, B., Gastaldelli, A., Pratipanawatr, T., Berria, R., Pratipanawatr, W., Bajaj, M., Mandarino, L., DeFronzo, R., Cusi, K. (2003). A sustained increase in plasma free fatty acids impairs secretion in nondiabetic subjects genetically predisposed to develop Type 2 Diabetes. *Diabetes, 52*:2461-2474.

Keenan, M. J., Janes, M., Robert, J., Martin, R. J., Raggio, A. M., McCutcheon, K. L., Pelkman, C., Tulley, R., Goita, M., Durham, H.A., Zhou, J., Senevirathne, R.N. (2013). Resistant starch from high amylose maize (HAM-RS2) reduces body fat and increases gut bacteria in ovariectomized (OVX) rats. *Obesity, 21*(5), 981-984.

Keenan, M. J., Zhou, J., McCutcheon, K. L., Raggio, A. M., Bateman, H. G., Todd, E., Jones, C.K., Tulley, R.T., Melton, S., Martin, R. J., Hegsted, M. (2006). Effects of resistant starch, A non-digestible fermentable fiber, on reducing body fat. *Obesity, 14*(9), 1523-1534.

Klosterbuer, A.S., Thomas, W., Slavin, J.L. (2012). Resistant starch and pullulan reduce postprandial glucose, insulin, and GLP-1, but have no effect on satiety in healthy humans. *Journal of Agricultural and Food Chemistry, 60*(48), 11929-11934.

Korus, J., Witczak, M., Ziobro, R., Juszczak, L. (2009). The impact of resistant starch on gluten-free dough and bread. *Food Hydrocolloids, 23,* 988-995.

Leszczyñski, W. (2004). Resistant starch-classification, structure, production. *Polish Journal of Food and Nutrition Sciences, 13*(54), 37-50.

Lin, H. V., Frassetto, A., Kowalik Jr, E. J., Nawrocki, A. R., Lu, M. M., Kosinski, J. R., Hubert, J.A., Szeto, D., Yao, X., Forrest, G., Forrest, G., Marsh, D.J. (2012). Butyrate and propionate protect against diet-induced obesity and regulate gut hormones via free fatty acid receptor 3-independent mechanisms. *PLoS One, 7*(4), e35240. doi:10.1371/journal.pone.0035240

Maki, K. C., Pelkman, C. L., Finocchiaro, E. T., Kelley, K. M., Lawless, A. L., Schild, A. L., & Rains, T. M. (2012). Resistant starch from high-amylose maize increases insulin sensitivity in overweight and obese men. *The Journal of Nutrition, 142*(4), 717-723.

Maljaars, P., Peters, H., Mela, D., & Masclee, A. (2008). Ileal brake: A sensible food target for appetite control. A review. *Physiology & Behavior, 95*(3), 271-281.

Maziarz, M., Sherrard, M., Juma, S., Prasad, C., Imrhan, V., & Vijayagopal, P. (2012). Sensory characteristics of high-amylose maize-resistant starch in three food products. *Food Science & Nutrition, 1*(2), 117-124.

Maziarz, M. P. (2013). Role of fructans and resistant starch in diabetes care. *Diabetes Spectrum, 26*(1), 35-39.

Maziarz, M., Juma, S., Imrhan, V., Prasad, C., Vijayagopal, P. (2014). *High-amylose maize resistant starch type 2 (HAM-RS2) influences satiety peptides and body composition in overweight adults*. Manuscript in preparation.

McCleary, B.V., Sloane, N., Draga, A., Lazewska, I. (2013). Measurement of total dietary fiber using AOAC method 2009.01 (AACC International Approved Method 32-45.01): Evaluation and updates. *Cereal Chemistry, 90*(4), 396-414.

Mermelstein, N.H. (2009). Analyzing for resistant starch. *Food Technology, 4*, 80-84.

Muir, J. G., Lu, Z. X., Young, G. P., Cameron-Smith, D., Collier, G. R., & O'Dea, K. (1995). Resistant starch in the diet increases breath hydrogen and serum acetate in human subjects. *The American Journal of Clinical Nutrition, 61*(4), 792-799.

Murphy, K. G., & Bloom, S. R. (2006). Gut hormones and the regulation of energy homeostasis. *Nature, 444*(7121), 854-859.

Murphy, M., Douglass, J., Birkett, A. (2008). Resistant starch intakes in the United States. *Journal of the American Dietetic Association, 108*(1), 67-78. doi:10.1016/j.jada.2007.10.012.

Neary, N. M., Small, C. J., Druce, M. R., Park, A. J., Ellis, S. M., Semjonous, N. M., Dakin, C.L., Flipsson, K., Wang, F., Kent, A.S., Frost, G.S., Ghatei, M.A., Bloom, S.R. (2005). Peptide YY3–36 and glucagon-like peptide-17–36 inhibit food intake additively. *Endocrinology, 146*(12), 5120-5127.

Nichenametla, S.N., Weidauer, L.A., Wey, H.E., Beare, T.M., Specker, B.L., Dey, M. (2014). Resistant starch type 4-enriched diet lowered blood cholesterols and improved body composition in a double blind controlled cross-over intervention. *Molecular Nutrition and Food Research, 00*, 1-5.

Noronha, N., O'Riordan, E.D., O'Sullivan, M. (2007). Replacement of fat with functional fibre in imitation cheese. *International Dairy Journal, 17*, 1073-1082.

Nugent, A. P. (2005). Health properties of resistant starch. *Nutrition Bulletin, 30,* 27-54.

Ozturk, S., Koksel, H. (2014). Production and characterisation of resistant starch and its utilisation as a food ingredient: A review. *Quality Assurance and Safety of Crops and Foods, 6*(3), 335-346.

Phillips, J., Muir, J. G., Birkett, A., Lu, Z. X., Jones, G. P., O'Dea, K., & Young, G. P. (1995). Effect of resistant starch on fecal bulk and fermentation-dependent events in humans. *The American Journal of Clinical Nutrition, 62*(1), 121-130.

Ritter, R. C. (2004). Gastrointestinal mechanisms of satiation for food. *Physiology & Behavior, 81*(2), 249-273.

Roberfroid, M., Gibson, G. R., Hoyles, L., McCartney, A. L., Rastall, R., Rowland, I., Wolvers, D., Watzl, B., Szajewska, H., Stahl, B., Guarner, F., Respondek, F., Whelan, K., Coxam, V., Davicco, M.J., Leotoing, L., Wittrant, Y., Delzenne, N.M., Cani, P.D., Neyrink, A.M., Meheust, A. (2010). Prebiotic effects: Metabolic and health benefits. *British Journal of Nutrition, 104*(S2), S1-S63.

Roberts, J., Jones, G.P., Gibbons, C., Birkett, A.M. (2004). Resistant starch in the Australian Diet. *Nutrition & Dietetics: The Journal of the Dietitian Association of Australia, 61*(2), 98-104.

Robertson, M. D. (2012). Dietary-resistant starch and glucose metabolism. *Current Opinion in Clinical Nutrition & Metabolic Care, 15*(4), 362-367.

Robertson, M. D., Wright, J. W., Loizon, E., Debard, C., Vidal, H., Shojaee-Moradie, F., Umpleby, A. M. (2012). Insulin-sensitizing effects on muscle and adipose tissue after dietary fiber intake in men and women with metabolic syndrome. *Journal of Clinical Endocrinology & Metabolism, 97*(9), 3326-3332.

Robertson, M. D., Bickerton, A. S., Dennis, A. L., Vidal, H., & Frayn, K. N. (2005). Insulin-sensitizing effects of dietary resistant starch and effects on skeletal muscle and adipose tissue metabolism. *The American Journal of Clinical Nutrition, 82*(3), 559-567.

Robertson, M., Currie, J., Morgan, L., Jewell, D., & Frayn, K. (2003). Prior short-term consumption of resistant starch enhances postprandial insulin sensitivity in healthy subjects. *Diabetologia, 46*(5), 659-665.

Sajilata, M.G., Singhal, R.S., Kulkarni, P.R. (2006). Resistant Starch - A review. *Comprehensive Reviews in Food Science and Food Safety*, *5*, 1-17.

Sanz, T., Salvador, A., Fiszman, S. (2008). Resistant starch (RS) in battered fried products: functionality and high-fibre benefit. *Food Hydrocolloids, 22*, 543-549.

Sharma, A., Yadav, B. S., & Ritika. (2008). Resistant starch: Physiological roles and food applications. *Food Reviews International, 24*(2), 193-234.

Shen, L., Keenan, M. J., Martin, R. J., Tulley, R. T., Raggio, A. M., McCutcheon, K. L., & Zhou, J. (2008). Dietary resistant starch increases hypothalamic POMC expression in rats. *Obesity, 17*(1), 40-45.

Skurk, T., Alberti-Huber, C., Herder, C., Hauner, H. (2007). Relationship between adipocyte size and adipokine expression and secretion. *Journal of Clinical Endorinology and Metabolism, 92*(3), 1023-1033.

Tharanathan, R. N. (2002). Food-derived carbohydrates-structural complexity and functional diversity. *Critical Reviews in Biotechnology, 22*(1), 65-84.

Tolhurst, G., Heffron, H., Lam, Y. S., Parker, H. E., Habib, A. M., Diakogiannaki, E., Cameron, J., Grosse, J., Reimann, F., Gribble, F. M. (2012). Short-chain fatty acids stimulate glucagon-like peptide-1 secretion via the G-Protein–Coupled receptor FFAR2. *Diabetes, 61*(2), 364-371.

Topping, D. L., & Clifton, P. M. (2001). Short-chain fatty acids and human colonic function: Roles of resistant starch and nonstarch polysaccharides. *Physiological Reviews, 81*(3), 1031-1064.

Willis, H. J., Eldridge, A. L., Beiseigel, J., Thomas, W., & Slavin, J. L. (2009). Greater satiety response with resistant starch and corn bran in human subjects. *Nutrition Research, 29*(2), 100-105.

Wong, J. M., de Souza, R., Kendall, C. W., Emam, A., & Jenkins, D. J. (2006). Colonic health: Fermentation and short chain fatty acids. *Journal of Clinical Gastroenterology, 40*(3), 235-243.

Xiong, Y., Miyamoto, N., Shibata, K., Valasek, M. A., Motoike, T., Kedzierski, R. M., & Yanagisawa, M. (2004). Short-chain fatty acids stimulate leptin production in adipocytes through the G protein-coupled receptor GPR41. *Proceedings of the National Academy of Sciences of the United States of America, 101*(4), 1045-1050.

Zhou, J., Martin, R.J., Tulley, R.T., Raggio, A.M., Shen, L., Lissy, E., McCutcheon, K., Keenan, M.J. (2009). Failure to ferment dietary resistant starch in specific mouse models of obesity results in no body fat loss. *Journal of Agriculture and food Chemistry, 57*(19), 8844-8851.

Zhou, J., Martin, R. J., Tulley, R. T., Raggio, A. M., McCutcheon, K. L., Shen, L., Danna, S.C., Tripathy, S., Hegsted, M., Keenan, M. J. (2008). Dietary resistant starch upregulates total GLP-1 and PYY in a sustained day-long manner through fermentation in rodents. *American Journal of Physiology-Endocrinology and Metabolism, 295*(5), E1160-E1166.

In: Dietary Fiber
Editor: Marvin E. Clemens
ISBN: 978-1-63463-655-1
© 2015 Nova Science Publishers, Inc.

Chapter 2

Role of Dietary Fibers on Health of the Gastro-Intestinal System and Related Types of Cancer

Raquel de Pinho Ferreira Guiné*
CI&DETS Research Centre and Department of Food Industry,
Polytechnic Institute of Viseu, ESAV, Quinta da Alagoa, Viseu, Portugal

Abstract

Dietary fibers are classified into water soluble or insoluble, and most plant foods include in their composition variable amounts of a mixture of soluble and insoluble fibers. This soluble or insoluble nature of fiber is related to its physiological effects. Insoluble fibers are characterized by high porosity, low density and the ability to increase fecal bulk, and act by facilitating intestinal transit, thus reducing the exposure to carcinogens in the colon and therefore acting as protectors against colon cancer. The influence of soluble fiber in the digestive tract includes its ability to retain water and form gels as well as a role as a substrate for fermentation of colon bacteria. However, the viscous soluble polysaccharides can delay digestion and compromise in some degree the absorption of nutrients from the gut.

Dietary fibers have an impact on all aspects of gut physiology and are a vital part of a healthy diet. Diets rich in dietary fiber have a protective effect against diseases such as hemorrhoids and some chronic diseases as well as in decreasing the incidence of various types of cancer, including colorectal, prostate and breast cancer.

The dietary fibers are among the most attractive and studied themes in nutrition and public health in the past decades, and therefore many epidemiological studies have been developed to evaluate the effects of fibers on several aspects of human health.

The current trend is towards diets rich in dietary fiber since these are implicated in the maintenance and/or improvement of health. However, despite the beneficial effects, there is also evidence of some negative effects associated with fiber consumption. For example, fiber can produce phytobenzoates, which can induce a decrease in the absorption and digestion of proteins. On the other hand, some fibers may inhibit the activity of pancreatic enzymes that digest carbohydrates, lipids and proteins.

* Corresponding author: E-mail: raquelguine@esav.ipv.pt.

Furthermore, fibers can interfere, although not strongly, with the absorption of some vitamins and minerals like calcium, iron, zinc and copper.

1. Nature of Dietary Fibers

The definition of dietary fiber is not unanimous, and a diversity of definitions can be found. While some are based on their physiological effects, others rely upon the analytical methods used to isolate and quantify them (Slavin, 2003).

Food fibers have been subject for much discussion among the scientific community over the last decades and there is still no international consensus on the definition of dietary fiber, or even a unique and precise methodology for its determination (Rodríguez et al., 2006).

According to Almeida and Afonso (1997) fiber is a generic terms that comprises a complex set of substances that include cellulose, hemicelluloses, pectins, gums, mucilages and lignin.

The American Association of Cereal Chemists in 2001 (AACC, 2001), defined dietary fiber as "the edible parts of plants or analogous carbohydrates that are resistant to digestion and absorption in the human small intestine with complete or partial fermentation in the large intestine. Dietary fiber includes polysaccharides, oligosaccharides, lignin, and associated plant substances" (Hong et al., 2012).

The Food and Nutrition Board proposed in 2001 two definitions, distinguishing dietary fiber from added fiber. According to those definitions, the first consists of nondigestible carbohydrates and lignin that are intrinsic and intact in plants, while the second consists of isolated, nondigestible carbohydrates that have beneficial physiological effects in humans. In this way, total fiber should account for the sum of dietary fiber plus added fiber (Slavin, 2003). These definitions were also adapted by the U. S. Institute of Medicine in 2002 and 2005 (IM, 2002). Also the Agence Française de Sécurité Sanitaire des Aliments proposed a definition for fiber in 2002 (AFSSA, 2002) and in 2006 definitions of dietary fiber were suggested from international organizations, namely: the Codex Alimentarius Commission (CAC, 2006) and Health Council of The Netherlands (HCN, 2006).

According to Slavin (2008), dietary fiber corresponds mainly to polysaccharides stored in the cell wall of plants that cannot be hydrolyzed by human digestive enzymes. In 2008 the Codex Commission on Nutrition and Foods for Special Dietary Uses (CCNFSDU) defined dietary fiber as carbohydrate polymers with ten or more monomeric units, which are not hydrolysed by endogenous enzymes in small intestine of human beings (Kendall et al., 2010). The European Commission in 2008 proposed a similar definition (Mann and Cummings, 2009). Yet, another definition that was derived by the Dietary Reference Intake (DRI) deliberations, divides fiber into three categories, namely dietary fiber, which includes wheat and oat bran, functional fiber, that includes resistant starches and total fiber, which is the sum of both (Kendall et al., 2010).

Dietary fibers can be classified into soluble or insoluble, according to their solubility in water (Elleuch et al., 2011). Most plant foods are formed by a mixture of soluble and insoluble fibers (Almeida and Afonso, 1997). Cellulose and lignin are called insoluble fiber or unfermentable because they do not dissolve in water or are metabolized by intestinal bacteria. This insoluble fiber is the structural part of plants. Contrarily, pectins, gums and mucilages exist within and around the plant cells. They are water soluble (acquiring a gel-like structure) and fermentable by colonic bacteria being called soluble or fermentable fiber (Almeida and Afonso, 1997).

The nature of the soluble and insoluble fiber is associated with differences in technological functionality and physiological effects (Elleuch et al., 2011). Insoluble fibers are characterized by high porosity, low density and the ability to increase fecal bulk. Their main task is to facilitate intestinal transit, thus reducing exposure to carcinogens in the colon and also decreasing the probability of occurrence of cancer (Elleuch et al., 2011).

Soluble fibers are characterized by the ability to increase viscosity and reduce the glycemic response and the levels of cholesterol in the blood stream. The influence of soluble fiber in the digestive tract is related to its ability to retain water and form gels and also by its role as a substrate for fermentation of bacteria in the colon (Escott-Stump et al., 2013). The soluble fraction acts as an emulsifier, providing good texture and good flavor. Besides, it is easier to incorporate into processed foods (Elleuch et al., 2011). However, the viscous soluble polysaccharides can hinder digestion and absorption of nutrients from the gut (Guillon and Champ, 2000). Among the soluble fibers are oat bran, barley bran and psyllium, associated with claims for lowering blood lipid levels, whereas wheat bran and other more insoluble fibers are typically linked to laxation (Slavin, 2008).

Dietary fiber was divided into soluble and insoluble fiber in an attempt to assign physiologic effects to different chemical types of fiber, however, the Institute of Medicine report and the National Academy of Sciences Panel on the Definition of Dietary Fiber recommended that these terms should not be used (Slavin, 2008, 2005).

2. The Dietary Fibers in the Diet

The human diets have been changing during the past decades, including increasing amounts of refined grains, meats, added fats and sugars and in opposition less vegetable proteins and low fiber intake (Hall et al., 2010; Kendall et al., 2010; O'Neil et al., 2010). It is recognized that diets low in fiber are frequently also poor in some essential micronutrients and high in sugars, salt, rapidly digested starches and fats (Mann and Cummings, 2009).

This trend to change the diet associated with factors such as cigarette smoking or a sedentary lifestyle due to lack of physical activity, is largely responsible for the increasing incidence of obesity and chronic diseases including type 2 diabetes, heart disease and cancer (Kendall et al., 2010; Mann and Cummings, 2009).

Increasing consumption of dietary fiber in food such as fruits, vegetables, whole grains, and legumes is critical for fighting the epidemic of obesity found in developed countries (Slavin, 2003). As reported by Sardinha et al. (2014) studies in Europe and in the United States have shown that the consumption of dietary fiber from different sources had a positive effect on weight loss and waist circumference reduction (Du et al., 2010; O'Neil et al., 2010). The effects of fiber consumption vary according to their solubility and chemical structure, and are manifested over appetite regulation, energy intake and body weight. However, the mechanisms involved in these relations are still to be fully understood (Wanders et al., 2011).

It is the position of the American Dietetic Association (ADA) that the public should consume adequate amounts of dietary fiber from a variety of plant foods (Marlett et al., 2002). The protective role of consumption of fiber-rich foods, including whole grain cereals, fruits and vegetables, on chronic diseases is well documented in the scientific literature (Chuang et al., 2012; Eshak et al., 2010; Kendall et al., 2010).

According to the World Health Organization (WHO, 2004), public interest in healthy eating has increased due to the high incidence of several human health disorders. In this way, there has been an increasing demand for healthy foods (Tudoran et al., 2009).

Food manufacturers use a large variety of dietary fiber ingredients either for technological or physiological purposes, improving textural properties or providing potential health benefits (Hall et al., 2010). Specific dietary fiber supplements, embraced as nutriceuticals or functional foods, are however, a still unknown way to influence modern diets (Wasan and Goodlad, 1996).

3. The Role of Dietary Fibers in Human Health

Dietary fibers have an impact on all aspects of gut physiology and are a vital part of a healthy diet (Brownlee, 2011). Studies have demonstrated that different sources of fiber can have different metabolic and physiological effects. Some of the beneficial physiological effects of dietary fibers include laxation as well as blood cholesterol and glucose attenuation (AACC, 2001).

Dietary fiber includes a diversity of macromolecules exhibiting a large variety of physical-chemical properties. Amongst these, the viscosity and ion exchange capacity are the main contributors to metabolic effects such as glucose and lipid metabolisms, whereas fermentation pattern, bulking effect and particle size are strongly involved on the colonic function (Guillon and Champ, 2000).

Dietary fiber presents the capacity to exchange many cations, and particularly some toxic cations, thus helping to excrete them with the feces. Furthermore, it can also absorb some of the harmful substances which play a role in disease prevention (Hong et al., 2012).

The dietary fibers represented one of the most attractive themes in nutrition and public health for some decades, thus originating a large number of epidemiological studies at the physiological, analytical and technical levels. Great advances were achieved in relation to the causes of several diseases, especially those connected to the large intestine or diabetes, and some targets valuable for defining a healthy diet were achieved (Cummings et al., 2004).

The scientific evidence that vegetables, fruits, and whole grains reduce the risk of chronic diseases is presently established, being this much attributed to the role of dietary fiber in the prevention of such diseases, as evidenced by many scientific studies (Kendall et al., 2010; Ludwig et al., 1999; Nayga, 1996).

Diseases of public health significance such as obesity, cardiovascular disease, type 2 diabetes or constipation can be fairly prevented or even treated by an adequate consumption of fiber rich foods throughout the lifecycle, from childhood to senior age (Slavin, 2003).

O'Neil et al. (2010) investigated the association of whole grain consumption with prevalence of overweight/obesity in adults. Their results confirm that those who consumed higher amounts of whole grains had lower body weight. Based on available data, Slavin (2008) stated that daily fiber intake of 20 to 27 g/day from whole foods or up to 20 g from supplements may help in weight control.

Diets rich in dietary fiber, mainly from fruits, green vegetables and legumes, have a protective effect against diseases such as arteriosclerosis, as well as other diseases, including cardiovascular disease, by reducing cholesterol levels and blood pressure (Rosamond, 2002). Experimental studies have associated dietary fiber with a favorable influence on cardiovascular risk factors, reduced risk of coronary heart disease, and significant lowering of total and LDL cholesterol (Mann and Cummings, 2009). The fibers have a great capacity to reduce serum cholesterol concentrations, particularly the soluble fraction (Gray, 2006). Dietary fiber intake, either from whole foods or supplements, may lower blood pressure, improve serum lipid levels, and reduce indicators of inflammation for daily intakes of 12 to 33 g when from whole foods or up to 42.5 g fiber when from supplements (Slavin, 2008).

Studies have demonstrated that high intakes of fiber are associated with reduced risk of type 2 diabetes lowering blood glucose and insulin levels (Mann and Cummings, 2009). Therefore, a diet rich in fiber (especially of the soluble type) will be beneficial in terms of glycemic control, as these food components often have a low glycemic index (Saldanha, 1999). According to Slavin (2008), diets providing 30 to 50 g fiber per day from whole food sources consistently produce lower serum glucose levels compared to a low-fiber diet. However, for fiber from supplements, dosages of 10 to 29 g/day may produce benefit in terms of glycemic control.

Fiber has significant physiological effects in the gut and, in addition, through fermentation, largely determines bowel function (Cummings et al., 2004). Experimental investigations demonstrate the effects of fiber on gut transit, stool weights, bile acid metabolism, intraluminal pressures and fermentation by colonic microflora (Mann and Cummings, 2009). Since fiber is not digested and absorbed in the small intestine, it can have a laxative effect (Slavin, 2008). Furthermore, a high-fiber diet is standard therapy for diverticular disease of the colon and may improve symptoms in patients with inflammatory bowel disease like Crohn's disease and ulcerative colitis (Slavin, 2008). Also Rodríguez et al. (2006) reported beneficial effects of dietary fiber on hemorrhoids.

Schatzkin et al. (2008) conducted a prospective study about the effects of dietary fiber on small intestinal cancer and concluded that the fiber intake was inversely associated with gastrointestinal cancers. Besides, fibre has also been associated with the decrease in the incidence of various types of cancer, including colorectal, prostate and breast cancer (Beecher, 1999; Bobek et al., 2000; Jiménez-Escrig et al., 2001; Ludwig et al., 1999; Park et al., 2009; Zhang et al., 2011).

The current trend is towards diets that include a greater amount of plant foods as these are implicated in the maintenance and/or improvement of health (Rodríguez et al., 2006). However, despite the beneficial effects mentioned above, there is also evidence of some negative health effects resulting from the intake of fiber. For example, fiber can produce phytobenzoates, which can induce a decrease in the absorption and digestion of proteins (Martinho et al., 2013). On the other hand, some fibers may inhibit the activity of pancreatic enzymes that digest carbohydrates, lipids and proteins (Harris and Ferguson, 1999). Furthermore, fibers can interfere, although not strongly, with the absorption of some vitamins and minerals like calcium, iron, zinc and copper (Hernández et al., 1995). However, it is unlikely that healthy adults who consume dietary fiber within the recommended dosages have problems relatively to nutrient absorption (Slavin, 2008). Besides, although typically dietary fibers are thought to decrease mineral absorption, fibers such as inulin, oligosaccharides, resistant starch or others, have been found to enhance mineral absorption, particularly for calcium (Slavin, 2008).

Another eventual negative effect of fiber ingestion is that the fermentation of dietary fiber by anaerobic bacteria in the large intestine produces gases, which may be related to complaints of distention or flatulence.

3.1. Dietary Fibers and Bowel Function

The physiological effects of fiber depend primarily on its physical properties and not so much on the chemical composition. The main physical properties that influence function are rheological properties of the water-soluble component, surface characteristics of the water-insoluble component and the properties of the hydrated complex, i.e., viscosity, water-holding capacity, cation exchange, organic acid adsorption (particularly bile acids), gel filtration and particle size distribution (Bosaeus, 2004).

The effects of fiber in the stomach and small intestine depend largely on the physical properties of the fiber source, since fibers with different physical characteristics affect gastrointestinal motility and transit times in different ways (Hillemeier, 1995; Vincent et al., 1995). Increased viscosity leads to delayed gastric emptying and thus delayed delivery of stomach contents into the small intestine, besides influencing absorption in the small intestine (Bosaeus, 2004).

Effects of fiber on the large intestine are mediated particularly through fermentation (Bosaeus, 2004). A major role of fiber is to provide a substrate for fermentation in the colon and stimulation of microbial growth. Colonic bacteria are important for fecal bulking, estimated to be up to 50% of fecal solids in subjects eating Western diets. Bacteria contain about 80% water and can resist dehydration, and thus are an important to the water-holding capacity of feces (Bosaeus, 2004; Cummings, 1984).

The microbial fermentation of fiber in the colon originates gases such as carbon dioxide, hydrogen and methane, which when trapped in the intestinal contents can result in an increase in stool volume, thus decreasing transit time (Bosaeus, 2004). The soluble fibers, that are more extensively degraded, primarily induce an increase in microbial mass and gas production, thus increasing fecal bulk. The insoluble fibers, usually less extensively degraded, retain their water-holding capacity, thus increasing stool bulk and stimulating colonic motility diminishing transit time (Bosaeus, 2004).

Some soluble nondigestible carbohydrates such as fructo-oligosaccharides, which are easily and rapidly fermented, have been shown to increase the number of bifidobacteria in feces, which is postulated to be beneficial for colonic health (Gibson and Roberfroid, 1995; Van Loo et al., 1999).

Increased fiber intake will generally increase stool weight, depending on the fiber source. The contributions of this increase from an elevated bacterial mass, fecal water and undigested fiber also vary markedly with the type of fiber (Cummings, 1984). Increased fiber particle size results in increased fecal output. Large particles are more slowly degraded, and thus to a larger extent expelled in feces. Indigestible plastic particles cut to the same size as coarse wheat bran flakes induce a comparable increase in stool weight (Bosaeus, 2004).

Rye bread and other rye products rich in fiber have shown to improve bowel function by increasing fecal weight and fecal frequency, and by shortening intestinal transit time, decrease the concentration of secondary bile acids and increase the concentration of plasma enterolactone (Gråsten et al., 2007, 2000; McIntosh et al., 2003).

At first fiber effects on intestinal function were associated to the resistance to digestion and retention of water in the fiber matrix, resulting in increased bulk and stimulation of colonic motility. However, presently it is understood that this is not the only mechanism and it was observed that fibers with high water-holding capacity *in vitro* have less effect on stool weight (Cummings, 1984). Water-holding capacity appears to be related to solubility as well as the rate of degradation by colonic micro flora. Hence, rapidly degraded fibers tend to have less effect on fecal weight (Bourquin et al., 1996). Almost all fibers are degraded to a greater or lesser extent in the colon, but certain fibers, e.g., the cellulosic fraction, survive digestion to a greater extent than non-cellulosic polysaccharides.

Intestinal transit time is reduced by increased bulk in the colon due to undigested fiber residue and microbial proliferation, resulting in decreased water absorption. Hence, fecal water and weight increases. Inert plastic particles given as bran-like flakes can also induce reduction in transit time and increased stool weight (Lewis and Heaton, 1999, 1997).

Approximately 20% of the world's population experiences functional bowel disorder including constipation and diverticulitis, and one of the most common therapeutic tools in those diseases is an oral intake of dietary fiber. Dietary fiber supplementation in sufficient daily dosages (20–30 g/day) can decrease gut transit time and improve bowel movement frequency (Cook et al., 1990; Ford and Talley, 2012; Occhipinti and Smith, 2012; Park and Jhon, 2009)

Constipation is a problem of the large intestine, and is a symptom rather than a disease, characterized by a low bowel frequency (e.g., <3/week), irregular stool expulsion, difficulties in defecation requiring straining, painful defecations, hard, dry stool consistency, a feeling of incomplete rectal evacuation and passing of abnormally small stools (e.g., <50 g/day). However, this is largely dependent on the person, since it is quite difficult to define normal bowel habits. Constipation can be due to a wide variety of diseases such as: organic bowel disorders with obstruction or motility disturbances, anal and pelvic disorders, neurological disease, metabolic and endocrine disorders. Still, it can also occur as a side-effect of many drugs or be due to dehydration or immobilization. Constipation can also occur in the absence of organic causes (chronic idiopathic constipation), associated with factors such as lack of exercise, denied bowel action, low fiber intake, disrupted lifestyle (e.g., long-distance travel, admission to hospital) or personality factors (Borum, 2001; Thompson, 2000; Wald, 2007).

Impaired bowel function, particularly constipation, is a common complaint of ill or inactive elderly people (Yen et al., 2011). Gastrointestinal function can also be compromised in children with a variety of disorders (Khoshoo et al., 2010).

Many studies we conducted about the effects of various fiber sources in the prevention or treatment of constipation in different patient groups (Tramonte et al., 1997).

Yen et al. (2011) evaluated the long-term effects of isomalto-oligosaccharide supplementation on fecal micro flora, bowel function, and biochemical indicators of nutritional status in constipated elderly subjects. They concluded that supplementation into a low-fiber diet improved colonic micro flora profile and bowel movement and that these beneficial effects decreased after discontinuation of the administration of the fiber supplements.

Chen et al. (2000) observed that supplementation of fructo-oligosaccharides was able to alleviate constipation, increase stool weight and fecal hort-chain fatty acid concentrations without affecting plasma lipid concentrations in normolipidemic constipated elderly men.

Donowitz et al. (1995) presented a physiological definition of diarrhea as a stool weight of more than 200 g/day. In routine practice, it is difficult to measure stool weight, and therefore other clinical definitions tend to be used. These usually define diarrhea as a change in consistency of stools and/or an increased frequency of bowel movements, as this is almost always associated with an increase in fecal water. There is, however, no universal agreement on this, and many quantitative and qualitative definitions have been used, the most common perhaps being the passage of three or more loose or liquid stools per day (Bosaeus, 2004). Fiber administration may increase colonic sodium and water absorption, as mediated by short chain fatty acids produced by fermentation. Furthermore, fiber may also improve stool consistency by sequestering water from liquid stools. Nakao et al. (2002) concluded that the administration of soluble dietary fiber was useful for the treatment of diarrhea during enteral nutrition in elderly patients by controlling spontaneous, favorable bowel movement and by improving symptoms of small intestinal mucosal atrophy and normalizing the intestinal flora. Rushdi et al. (2004) investigated the efficacy of the polysaccharide soluble dietary fiber guar gum in controlling preexisting diarrhea, as a candidate prebiotic and its potential benefits in intensive care unit patients on enteral nutrition.

3.2. Dietary Fibers and Diverticular Disease

Colonic diverticulosis refers to small outpouchings from the colonic lumen due to mucosal herniation through the colonic wall at sites of vascular perforation. Diverticulitis occurs when the colonic diverticulum and surrounding tissues become inflamed, frequently as the result of obstruction by dietary products or stool. This pathology is associated with abnormal colonic motility and inadequate intake of dietary fiber. Diverticulosis is more frequent in developed countries and its prevalence increases with age. Most patients affected do not experience any symptoms but 10 to 20% of those affected can manifest clinical syndromes, mainly diverticulitis and diverticular haemorrhage (Stollman and Raskin, 2004; Van Duyn and Pivonka, 2000).

High-fiber diets, which help to increase stool bulk and moisture and reduce travel time through the gastrointestinal tract, provide substantial defense against the development of diverticulosis. Insoluble fiber may be the type of dietary fiber most responsible for this protective role (Van Duyn and Pivonka, 2000).

The geographic variability of diverticular disease and its correlation with a western diet seem to suggest its strong dependence on the diet. Painter and Burkitt (1971) defended that diverticulosis could be avoided by implementing dietary changes and they studied the transit times and stool weights from more than 1200 individuals in the UK and rural Uganda (Burkitt et al., 1972). While the UK patients, eating a low fiber diet, had transit times of about 80 h and mean stool weights of 110 g/day, the rural Ugandans, eating very high fiber diets, had transit times of 34 h and weights of more than 450 g/day. The longer transit time and smaller stool volumes were thought to increase intraluminal pressure, predisposing to diverticular herniation.

Fisher et al. (1985) investigated the relationship between consumption of dietary fiber and the development of diverticular disease of the colon in an *in vivo* model with rats. The study offered strong support to the hypothesis of human diverticular disease being due to fiber deficiency. 45% of rats on the lowest fiber diet developed diverticula compared with only 9% of those fed the highest fiber diet. Furthermore, effects of fiber on body weight, food intake, mineral levels, blood composition and properties, mortality, organ weights, and incidence of tumors and lesions were reported.

Wess et al. (1996), in another *in vivo* model, concluded that high fiber diets protected against collagen crosslinking and that was associated with reduced frequency of development of colonic diverticulosis.

Aldoori et al. (1994) identified an association between fiber from fruits and vegetables and a reduced risk of diverticulosis. However, this was not true for fiber from cereal sources. Aldoori et al. (1998) also found that insoluble fiber, particularly cellulose, was significantly associated with a decreased risk of developing diverticulosis among a large group of male individuals.

Cunningham and Marcason (2002) report that increasing the amount of fiber in the diet may reduce the symptoms of diverticulosis and prevent complications, and they also refer that insoluble fiber, especially the cellulose in fruits and vegetables, may be particularly important in preventing diverticulosis.

3.3. Dietary Fibers and Inflammatory Bowel Disease (IBD)

The inflammatory bowel disease (IBD) comprises the Crohn's disease (CD) and ulcerative colitis (UC). These pathologies have been known for over 50 years, but the reasons why affected individuals spend their lives with a chronic inflammatory process that relentlessly destroys their bowel remains a mystery. No single agent or distinct mechanism is the single responsible to explain all aspects of IBD, and several distinguishing factors are likely necessary to result in either CD or UC (Fiocchi, 1998). The geographical and temporal variation in the incidence of inflammatory bowel disease stands in the first place on the list of the 10 remaining mysteries of inflammatory bowel disease (Colombel et al., 2008; Sjöberg et al., 2014).

Crohn's disease is a chronic inflammatory bowel disease that can affect any part of the gastrointestinal tract. It usually involves the terminal ileum and proximal colon, and its etiology and pathogenesis id determined by both genetic and environmental factors (Loftus, 2004; Stange et al., 2006; Stefanelli et al., 2008; van Loo et al., 2012). This disease is commonly diagnosed at late adolescence and early adulthood, although it can also appear at all other ages. Still, most patients are diagnosed before the age of 40 years (van Loo et al., 2012).

Ananthakrishnan et al. (2013) suggest that increased dietary fiber intake, specifically from fruits, may have a protective effect on development of CD but not on UC. They postulate two potential mechanism, including changes in the composition of the microbiota and increased fermentation of fiber from fruit into short chain fatty acids leading to decreased proinflammatory mediators, as well as increased activation of the aryl hydrocarbon receptor leading to improved protection against environmental insults (Kaplan, 2013; Stein and Cohen,

2014). However, Stein and Cohen (2014) alert that high-fiber diets are to be avoided in patients with CD, and particularly in those with ileal disease, because a high dietary fiber intake can lead to bowel obstructions. Furthermore, they state that misunderstanding the potential benefits of high fiber intake could have a negative impact for patients with CD.

A link between diet and IBD seems logical because it affects the very site of nutrient absorption. Nutritional deficiencies in IBD are well documented, particularly that of zinc in CD with associated immunologic dysfunction (Ainley et al., 1991).

The effectiveness of elemental or special diets in reducing the symptoms or inducing remission of CD has been proposed but not universally accepted. A controlled trial was conducted by O'Moráin et al. (1984) in which 21 patients acutely ill with exacerbations of Crohn's disease were randomised to receive either prednisolone 0.75 mg/kg/day or an elemental diet (Vivonex) for four weeks. Assessment at four and 12 weeks showed that the patients treated with the elemental diet had improved as much as or even more than the steroid treated group, thus allowing concluding that elemental diet is a safe and effective treatment for acute Crohn's disease.

In another study from Lochs et al. (1991) was compared the effect of enteral nutrition as the sole therapy of active Crohn's disease with drug treatment. In this case, the results showed that enteral nutrition was less effective than in treating active Crohn's disease.

Some data suggest that elemental diet may improve CD by reducing intestinal permeability, but it is not clear why nutritional therapies improve CD but not UC (Fiocchi, 1998; Teahon et al., 1991).

Suwannaporn et al. (2013) suggested that carbohydrates may provide an alternative therapeutic approach for a number of digestive health disorders including IBD, and conducted a study to characterize the tolerance and efficacy of low and high molecular weight konjac glucomannan hydrolysates within healthy volunteers and patients suffering from IBD and associated gut conditions. These conditions included constipation, Crohn's disease and ulcerative colitis. Their results showed that most patients experienced an improvement of their condition after consuming the hydrolysates. Furthermore, the use of the hydrolysates as a therapeutic agent or adjunct to standard treatments could prove a successful tool for the treatment of a range of disorders related to the intestinal health. Still, they alert that further studies are required to characterize more precisely the role of the carbohydrates.

Ulcers in the gastrointestinal tract could be divided into two common types according to location; ulcerative colitis (lower) and peptic ulcer (upper) (Awaad et al., 2013). Ulcerative colitis is a chronic inflammatory disorder of the colon that is characterized by alternating periods of flare-ups and quiescent disease. UC seems to result from an exaggerated intestinal host response against luminal bacteria or their components, and this is particularly true in genetically susceptible individuals. Also oxidative stress has been proposed to play a role in the pathophysiology of UC. This results from an excessive production of reactive oxygen species due to aberrant cellular metabolism and increased activation of phagocytic leucocytes in the inflamed colon (Hamer et al., 2010).

Peptic ulcer disease (PUD) is an illness that affects a considerable number of people worldwide and it develops when there is an imbalance between the "aggressive" and "protective" factors at the luminal surface of the epithelial cells. Aggressive factors include **Helicobacter pylori**, HCl, pepsins, nonsteroidal anti-inflammatory drugs, bile acids, ischemia, hypoxia, smoking and alcohol (Awaad et al., 2013; Kalant et al., 2006).

There is increasing interest in adding indigestible fibers to dietary products as a consequence of the several epidemiological studies that show protective effects of dietary fiber intake on intestinal inflammation, among other diseases. Short-chain fatty acids (mainly acetate, propionate and butyrate) are important end-products of luminal microbial fermentation of those fibers and have proved to help maintaining the colonic health and barrier function (Ajani et al., 2004; Hamer et al., 2010).

Studies have been conducted to examine the role of dietary factors in UC and how these influence the development of the disease. Epidemiological studies have examined the relationship between dietary intake and the onset of UC (Geerling et al., 2000; Jowett et al., 2004; Russel et al., 1998).

The studies about the effect of dietary fiber on UC are not always in agreement. For example, dietary fiber as a complement to standard treatment significantly improved the symptoms in a group of patients with UC (Hallert et al., 1991), but, on the other hand, in a non-randomised study comparing sulfasalazine with bran fiber there were more relapses for the patients taking bran (Davies and Rhodes, 1978).

Fernández-Bañares (1999) studied the efficacy and safety of *Plantago ovata* seeds (dietary fiber) as compared with mesalamine in maintaining remission in ulcerative colitis by means of a randomized clinical trial conducted with a total of 105 patients with ulcerative colitis who were in remission. They concluded that the dietary fiber might be as effective as mesalamine to maintain remission in ulcerative colitis.

Seidner et al. (2005) conducted a randomized controlled trial on an oral supplement enriched with fish oil, soluble fiber, and antioxidants for corticosteroid sparing in ulcerative colitis and their findings suggest that, attending the improvement in clinical response combined with a decreased requirement for corticosteroids, this enriched oral supplement can be a useful adjuvant therapy in patients suffering from UC.

Fujimori et al. (2009) conducted a randomized controlled trial on the efficacy of synbiotic versus probiotic or prebiotic treatment to improve the quality of life in patients with ulcerative colitis. They concluded that patients with UC on synbiotic therapy experienced better results than patients on probiotic or prebiotic treatment. These data suggest that synbiotic therapy (fibers plus microorganism) may have a synergistic effect in the treatment of UC.

3.4. Dietary Fibers and Gastro-Intestinal Related Types of Cancer

Oesophageal cancer is the eighth most common malignancy and the sixth leading cause of cancer-related deaths worldwide. However, the incidence of oesophageal cancer varies widely among different geographic areas (Ferlay et al., 2010; Tang et al., 2013). Scientific research suggests a possible protective effect of dietary fiber against the development of oesophageal cancer (Chen et al., 2002; Jessri et al., 2011). Also a few studies have investigated specific sources of fiber as having a protective role on this type of cancer (Tang et al., 2013; Terry et al., 2001; Wu et al., 2007).

Stomach cancer is the fourth most common cancer and the second leading cause of cancer deaths worldwide. There are about 880,000 new cases of stomach cancer, and about 650,000 people die of this disease each year, despite of the decrease in overall death rate from stomach cancer over the past decades owing to early detection and improvements in treatment (Brenner et al., 2009; Crew and Neugut, 2006; Han et al., 2013).

Although risk factors for squamous cell carcinoma of the esophagus and adenocarcinomas of the esophagus, gastric cardia, and other (noncardia) gastric sites have been identified, little is known about interactions among risk factors (Navarro Silvera et al., 2014).

It is believed that dietary factors play an important role in the prevention of gastric cancer, and among those undoubtedly that dietary fiber has received considerable interest. *In vitro* studies suggest that dietary fiber may prevent gastric cancer by acting as a nitrite scavenger, potentially countering the carcinogenic effects of N-nitroso compounds (Gonzalez and Riboli, 2010; Møller et al., 1988; Zhang et al., 2013). Also in vivo trials support the protective role of dietary fiber on stomach cancer. Zhang et al. (2013) studied the association between dietary fiber intake and gastric cancer risk by conducting a meta-analysis of case-control and cohort studies to analyze this association. Their results showed that dietary fiber intake was in fact inversely associated with gastric cancer risk. They hypothesized that the effect probably was independent of conventional risk factors. However, the trend of the protective association of dietary fiber was consistent among all studies.

Terry et al. (2001) examined data from a large-scale population-based case-control study of risk factors for adenocarcinoma of the gastric cardia carcinoma. Their results indicated an inverse association between intake of cereal fiber and risk of gastric cardia cancer.

Navarro Silvera et al. (2014) investigated the interactions of diet, other lifestyle, and medical factors with risks of subtypes of esophageal and gastric cancers. A review of the literature made by Thrift et al. (2012) showed that the regular fruit and vegetable intake is associated with a lower risk of developing cancer.

Reddy (1999) reported much evidence from scientific studies about the role of dietary fibers in protecting against colon cancer. Studies have demonstrated a reduced risk of colon cancer when populations with diets high in total fat switched to a diet high in total fiber and certain whole-grain foods. Case-control studies have shown convincingly the relationship between dietary fiber and colon cancer prevention. Furthermore, human dietary intervention studies have also indicated that the modifying effect of dietary fiber on bacterial enzymes involved in the production of putative colon tumor promoters depends on the type of fiber consumed. Dietary wheat bran, but not oat or corn bran, significantly decreased the levels of several tumor promoters in the colon, independent of stool bulk (Fuchs et al., 1999; Howe et al., 1992; Trock et al., 1990). On the other hand, studies conducted in animal models have demonstrated that the inhibitory effects of dietary fiber on the development of colonic neoplasms depend on the nature and source of the fiber. Also these studies revealed that wheat bran appears to inhibit colon tumor development more consistently than other dietary sources of fiber, such as oat and corn bran. Finally, dietary administration of phytic acid, high levels of which are present in wheat bran, showed to inhibit colon carcinogenesis (Reddy and Mori, 1981; Reddy et al., 1981).

The official recommendations of the American Gastroenterological Association (AGA) on the impact of dietary fiber on colon cancer occurrence were presented in a document released in 2000 (AGA, 2000). The position was approved by the Clinical Practice and Practice Economics Committee on September 25, 1999, and by the AGA Governing Board on November 15, 1999. The recommendations were that the available evidence at date from epidemiological, animal, and intervention studies did not unequivocally support the protective role of fiber against development of colorectal cancer (CRC). However, when the whole body of evidence from these studies is analyzed critically, the overall conclusion supports an inverse association between dietary fiber intake and CRC risk. However, the magnitude of CRC risk reduction and threshold level above which dietary fiber is associated with a significant degree of CRC risk reduction need to be more clearly defined.

Recent studies suggest that a high intake of fiber from cereals and high consumption of wholegrain foods is significantly associated with a reduced risk of colorectal cancer (Aune et al., 2011; Azuma et al., 2013; Ben et al., 2014; Ho et al., 1991; Khalid et al., 2014; Ma et al., 2013; Scharlau et al., 2009; Stein et al., 2012).

CONCLUSION

There is accumulated evidence on some of the benefits of dietary fiber for the health of the gastrointestinal system.

Fiber, particularly insoluble fiber, can help prevent constipation, by bulking up stools and keeping food moving through the digestive tract.

Some types of soluble fiber are considered prebiotics, i.e., they serve as food for the healthy bacteria that colonize the human intestine and therefore contribute for the increase in the numbers of such bacteria. These bacteria boost digestive health and might have far-reaching effects, perhaps improving the immune response and preventing allergy development.

Dietary fiber also has a beneficial effect on diverticulitis, a painful condition caused when pockets in the intestines rupture and become infected.

Irritable bowel syndrome can also be prevented and/or treated by the intake of dietary fibers such as those containing psyllium, guar gum, and methylcellulose. However, high-fiber wheat bran seems to worsen the symptoms.

A diet high in fiber has repeatedly shown benefits in preventing the types of cancer associated to the gastrointestinal tract (oesophageal, stomack, colorectal).

Finally, fiber's benefits aren't confined to digestive health and studies have demonstrated that healthy fiber can also lower cholesterol, promote healthy blood sugar levels, reduce the risk of cardiovascular disease, and help people lose weight or maintain a healthy weight.

ACKNOWLEDGMENT

The author would like to thank the valuable contribution of the reviewer of the present chapter: Prof. Maria João Barroca (PhD), Department of Chemical and Biological Engineering, Polytechnic Institute of Coimbra, Portugal.

REFERENCES

AACC, (2001). AACC Report: Dietary Fiber Technical Committee. The definition of dietary fiber. *Cereal Foods World*, *46*, 112–126.

AFSSA, (2002). Les fibres alimentaire: définitions, méthodes de dosage, allégations nutritionelles. Rapport du comité d'experts spécialisé nutrition humaine. Agence Française de Sécurité Sanitaire des Aliments, France.

AGA, (2000). American Gastroenterological Association medical position statement: Impact of dietary fiber on colon cancer occurrence. *Gastroenterology*, *118*, 1233–1234. doi:10.1016/S0016-5085(00)70376-3

Ainley, C., Cason, J., Slavin, B. M., Wolstencroft, R. A. & Thompson, R. P. (1991). The influence of zinc status and malnutrition on immunological function in Crohn's disease. *Gastroenterology*, *100*, 1616–1625.

Ajani, U. A., Ford, E. S. & Mokdad, A. H. (2004). Dietary fiber and C-reactive protein: findings from national health and nutrition examination survey data. *J. Nutr.*, *134*, 1181–1185.

Aldoori, W. H., Giovannucci, E. L., Rimm, E. B., Wing, A. L., Trichopoulos, D. V. & Willett, W. C. (1994). A prospective study of diet and the risk of symptomatic diverticular disease in men. *Am. J. Clin. Nutr.*, *60*, 757–764.

Aldoori, W. H., Giovannucci, E. L., Rockett, H. R., Sampson, L., Rimm, E. B. & Willett, W. C. (1998). A prospective study of dietary fiber types and symptomatic diverticular disease in men. *J. Nutr.*, *128*, 714–719.

Almeida, M. D. V. & Afonso, C. I. P. N. (1997). Princípios Básicos de Alimentação e Nutrição Princípios Básicos de Alimentação e Nutrição. Universidade Aberta, Lisbon, Portugal.

Ananthakrishnan, A. N., Khalili, H., Konijeti, G. G., Higuchi, L. M., de Silva, P., Korzenik, J. R., Fuchs, C. S., Willett, W. C., Richter, J. M. & Chan, A. T. (2013). A Prospective Study of Long-term Intake of Dietary Fiber and Risk of Crohn's Disease and Ulcerative Colitis. *Gastroenterology*, *145*, 970–977. doi:10.1053/j.gastro.2013.07.050

Aune, D., Chan, D. S. M., Lau, R., Vieira, R., Greenwood, D. C., Kampman, E. & Norat, T., (2011). Dietary fibre, whole grains, and risk of colorectal cancer: systematic review and dose-response meta-analysis of prospective studies. *BMJ*, 343, d6617–d6617. doi:10.1136/bmj.d6617

Awaad, A. S., El-Meligy, R. M. & Soliman, G. A. (2013). Natural products in treatment of ulcerative colitis and peptic ulcer. *Journal of Saudi Chemical Society*, *17*, 101–124. doi:10.1016/j.jscs.2012.03.002

Azuma, K., Osaki, T., Ifuku, S., Maeda, H., Morimoto, M., Takashima, O., Tsuka, T., Imagawa, T., Okamoto, Y., Saimoto, H. & Minami, S. (2013). Suppressive effects of cellulose nanofibers—made from adlay and seaweed—on colon inflammation in an inflammatory bowel-disease model. *Bioactive Carbohydrates and Dietary Fibre*, *2*, 65–72. doi:10.1016/j.bcdf.2013.09.006

Beecher, G. R. (1999). Phytonutrients' role in metabolism: effects on resistance to degenerative processes. *Nutr. Rev.*, *57*, S3–6.

Ben, Q., Sun, Y., Chai, R., Qian, A., Xu, B. & Yuan, Y. (2014). Dietary Fiber Intake Reduces Risk for Colorectal Adenoma: A Meta-analysis. *Gastroenterology*, *146*, 689–699.e6. doi:10.1053/j.gastro.2013.11.003

Bobek, P., Galbavý, Š. & Máriássyová, M. (2000). Effect of inulin on nutritional hypercholesterolemia and chemically induced precancerous lesions on rat colon. *Bulletin Potravinárskeho Výskumu*, *39*, 213–221.

Borum, M. L. (2001). Constipation: evaluation and management. *Prim. Care*, *28*, 577–590, vi.

Bosaeus, I. (2004). Fibre effects on intestinal functions (diarrhoea, constipation and irritable bowel syndrome). Clinical Nutrition Supplements, Effects and benefits of fibre in clinical practice. *Proceedings of a Consensus Conference.*, *1*, 33–38. doi:10.1016/j. clnu.2004.09.006

Bourquin, L. D., Titgemeyer, E. C. & Fahey, Jr. G. C. (1996). Fermentation of various dietary fiber sources by human fecal bacteria. *Nutrition Research*, *16*, 1119–1131. doi:10.1016/0271-5317(96)00116-9

Brenner, H., Rothenbacher, D. & Arndt, V. (2009). Epidemiology of stomach cancer. *Methods Mol. Biol.*, *472*, 467–477. doi:10.1007/978-1-60327-492-0_23

Brownlee, I. A. (2011). The physiological roles of dietary fibre. Food Hydrocolloids, *Dietary Fibre and Bioactive Polysaccharides*, *25*, 238–250. doi:10.1016/j.foodhyd.2009.11.013.

Burkitt, D.., Walker, A. R. & Painter, N. (1972). Effect of dietary fibre on stools and transit-times, and its role in the causation of disease. *The Lancet*, *300*, 1408–1411. doi:10.1016/S0140-6736(72)92974-1

CAC, (2006). Report of the 27th session of the Codex Committee on Nutrition and Foods for Special Dietary Uses, Bonn, Germany 21-25 November 2005. ALINORM 06/29/26. Codex Alimentarius Commission.

Chen, H., Tucker, K. L., Graubard, B. I., Heineman, E. F., Markin, R. S., Potischman, N. A., Russell, R. M., Weisenburger, D. D. & Ward, M. H. (2002). Nutrient intakes and adenocarcinoma of the esophagus and distal stomach. *Nutr Cancer*, *42*, 33–40. doi:10.1207/S15327914NC421_5

Chen, H. L., Lu, Y. H., Lin Jr, J. & Ko, L. Y. (2000). Effects of fructooligosaccharide on bowel function and indicators of nutritional status in constipated elderly men. *Nutrition Research*, *20*, 1725–1733. doi:10.1016/S0271-5317(00)00274-8

Chuang, S. C., Norat, T., Murphy, N., Olsen, A., Tjønneland, A., Overvad, K., Boutron-Ruault, M. C., Perquier, F., Dartois, L., Kaaks, R., Teucher, B., Bergmann, M. M., Boeing, H., Trichopoulou, A., Lagiou, P., Trichopoulos, D., Grioni, S., Sacerdote, C., Panico, S., Palli, D., Tumino, R., Peeters, P. H. M., Bueno-de-Mesquita, B., Ros, M. M., Brustad, M., Åsli, L.A., Skeie, G., Quirós, J. R., González, C. A., Sánchez, M. J., Navarro, C., Ardanaz Aicua, E., Dorronsoro, M., Drake, I., Sonestedt, E., Johansson, I., Hallmans, G., Key, T., Crowe, F., Khaw, K. T., Wareham, N., Ferrari, P., Slimani, N., Romieu, I., Gallo, V., Riboli, E. & Vineis, P. (2012). Fiber intake and total and cause-specific mortality in the European Prospective Investigation into Cancer and Nutrition cohort. *Am. J. Clin. Nutr.*, *96*, 164–174. doi:10.3945/ajcn.111.028415

Colombel, J. F., Watson, A. J. M. & Neurath, M. F. (2008). The 10 remaining mysteries of inflammatory bowel disease. *Gut*, *57*, 429–433. doi:10.1136/gut.2007.122192

Cook, I. J., Irvine, E. J., Campbell, D., Shannon, S., Reddy, S. N. & Collins, S. M. (1990). Effect of dietary fiber on symptoms and rectosigmoid motility in patients with irritable bowel syndrome. A controlled, crossover study. *Gastroenterology*, *98*, 66–72.

Crew, K. D. & Neugut, A. I. (2006). Epidemiology of gastric cancer. *World J. Gastroenterol.*, *12*, 354–362.

Cummings, J. H. (1984). Constipation, dietary fibre and the control of large bowel function. *Postgrad Med J*, *60*, 811–819.

Cummings, J. H., Edmond, L. M. & Magee, E. A. (2004). Dietary carbohydrates and health: do we still need the fibre concept? Clinical Nutrition Supplements, Effects and benefits of fibre in clinical practice. *Proceedings of a Consensus Conference.*, *1*, 5–17. doi:10.1016/j.clnu.2004.09.003

Cunningham, E. & Marcason, W. (2002). What Role Does Fiber Play in Diverticular Disease? *Journal of the American Dietetic Association*, *102*, 225. doi:10.1016/S0002-8223(02)90052-0

Davies, P. S. & Rhodes, J. (1978). Maintenance of remission in ulcerative colitis with sulphasalazine or a high-fibre diet: a clinical trial. *Br Med J*, *1*, 1524–1525.

Donowitz, M., Kokke, F. T. & Saidi, R. (1995). Evaluation of Patients with Chronic Diarrhea. *New England Journal of Medicine*, *332*, 725–729. doi:10.1056/NEJM199503163321107

Du, H., van der, A., D. L., Boshuizen, H. C., Forouhi, N. G., Wareham, N. J., Halkjaer, J., Tjønneland, A., Overvad, K., Jakobsen, M. U., Boeing, H., Buijsse, B., Masala, G., Palli, D., Sørensen, T. I. A., Saris, W. H. M. & Feskens, E. J. M. (2010). Dietary fiber and subsequent changes in body weight and waist circumference in European men and women. *Am. J. Clin. Nutr.*, *91*, 329–336. doi:10.3945/ajcn.2009.28191

Elleuch, M., Bedigian, D., Roiseux, O., Besbes, S., Blecker, C. & Attia, H. (2011). Dietary fibre and fibre-rich by-products of food processing: Characterisation, technological functionality and commercial applications: *A review. Food Chemistry*, *124*, 411–421. doi:10.1016/j.foodchem.2010.06.077

Escott-Stump, S., Mahan, K. L. & Raymond, J. L. (2013). Krause - Alimentos, Nutrição e Dietoterapia, 13th ed. Elsevier / medicina Nacionais, Brazil.

Eshak, E. S., Iso, H., Date, C., Kikuchi, S., Watanabe, Y., Wada, Y., Wakai, K., Tamakoshi, A. & JACC Study Group, (2010). Dietary fiber intake is associated with reduced risk of mortality from cardiovascular disease among Japanese men and women. *J. Nutr.*, *140*, 1445–1453. doi:10.3945/jn.110.122358

Ferlay, J., Shin, H., Bray, F., Forman, D., Mathers, C. & Parkin, D. (2010). Cancer incidence and mortality worldwide. International Agency for Research on Cancer, Lyon, France.

Fernández-Bañares, F., Hinojosa, J., Sánchez-Lombraña, J. L., Navarro, E., Martínez-Salmerón, J. F., García-Pugés, A., González-Huix, F., Riera, J., González-Lara, V., Domínguez-Abascal, F., Giné, J. J., Moles, J., Gomollón, F. & Gassull, M. A. (1999). Randomized clinical trial of Plantago ovata seeds (dietary fiber) as compared with mesalamine in maintaining remission in ulcerative colitis. *The American Journal of Gastroenterology*, *94*, 427–433. doi:10.1016/S0002-9270(98)00753-9

Fiocchi, C. (1998). Inflammatory bowel disease: Etiology and pathogenesis. *Gastroenterology*, *115*, 182–205. doi:10.1016/S0016-5085(98)70381-6

Fisher, N., Berry, C. S., Fearn, T., Gregory, J. A. & Hardy, J. (1985). Cereal dietary fiber consumption and diverticular disease: a lifespan study in rats. *Am. J. Clin. Nutr.*, *42*, 788–804.

Ford, A. C. & Talley, N. J. (2012). Irritable bowel syndrome. *BMJ*, *345*, e5836–e5836. doi:10.1136/bmj.e5836

Fuchs, C. S., Giovannucci, E. L., Colditz, G. A., Hunter, D. J., Stampfer, M. J., Rosner, B., Speizer, F. E. & Willett, W. C. (1999). Dietary Fiber and the Risk of Colorectal Cancer and Adenoma in Women. *New England Journal of Medicine*, *340*, 169–176. doi:10.1056/NEJM199901213400301

Fujimori, S., Gudis, K., Mitsui, K., Seo, T., Yonezawa, M., Tanaka, S., Tatsuguchi, A. & Sakamoto, C. (2009). A randomized controlled trial on the efficacy of synbiotic versus probiotic or prebiotic treatment to improve the quality of life in patients with ulcerative colitis. *Nutrition*, *25*, 520–525. doi:10.1016/j.nut.2008.11.017

Geerling, B. J., Dagnelie, P. C., Badart-Smook, A., Russel, M. G., Stockbrügger, R. W. & Brummer, R. J. (2000). Diet as a risk factor for the development of ulcerative colitis. *Am. J. Gastroenterol.*, *95*, 1008–1013. doi:10.1111/j.1572-0241.2000.01942.x

Gibson, G. R. & Roberfroid, M. B. (1995). Dietary modulation of the human colonic microbiota: introducing the concept of prebiotics. *J. Nutr.*, *125*, 1401–1412.

Gonzalez, C. A. & Riboli, E. (2010). Diet and cancer prevention: Contributions from the European Prospective Investigation into Cancer and Nutrition (EPIC) study. *Eur. J. Cancer*, *46*, 2555–2562. doi:10.1016/j.ejca.2010.07.025

Gråsten, S. M., Juntunen, K. S., Mättö, J., Mykkänen, O. T., El-Nezami, H., Adlercreutz, H., Poutanen, K. S. & Mykkänen, H. M. (2007). High-fiber rye bread improves bowel function in postmenopausal women but does not cause other putatively positive changes in the metabolic activity of intestinal microbiota. *Nutrition Research*, *27*, 454–461. doi:10.1016/j.nutres.2007.05.010

Gråsten, S. M., Juntunen, K. S., Poutanen, K. S., Gylling, H. K., Miettinen, T. A. & Mykkänen, H. M. (2000). Rye bread improves bowel function and decreases the concentrations of some compounds that are putative colon cancer risk markers in middle-aged women and men. *J. Nutr.*, *130*, 2215–2221.

Gray, J. (2006). Dietary fiber – definition, analysis, physiology & health. Internacional Life Sciences Institute, Belgium.

Guillon, F. & Champ, M. (2000). Structural and physical properties of dietary fibres, and consequences of processing on human physiology. *Food Research International*, *33*, 233–245. doi:10.1016/S0963-9969(00)00038-7

Hall, R. S., Baxter, A. L., Fryirs, C. & Johnson, S. K. (2010). Liking of health-functional foods containing lupin kernel fibre following repeated consumption in a dietary intervention setting. *Appetite*, *55*, 232–237. doi:10.1016/j.appet.2010.06.004

Hallert, C., Kaldma, M. & Petersson, B. G. (1991). Ispaghula husk may relieve gastrointestinal symptoms in ulcerative colitis in remission. *Scand. J. Gastroenterol.*, *26*, 747–750. doi:10.3109/00365529108998594

Hamer, H. M., Jonkers, D. M. A. E., Vanhoutvin, S. A. L. W., Troost, F. J., Rijkers, G., de Bruïne, A., Bast, A., Venema, K. & Brummer, R. J. M. (2010). Effect of butyrate enemas on inflammation and antioxidant status in the colonic mucosa of patients with ulcerative colitis in remission. *Clinical Nutrition*, *29*, 738–744. doi:10.1016/j.clnu.2010.04.002

Han, K. H., Hwang, I. C., Kim, S., Bae, J. M., Kim, Y. W., Ryu, K. W., Lee, J. H., Noh, J. H., Sohn, T. S., Shin, D. W. & Yun, Y. H. (2013). Factors Associated With Depression in Disease-Free Stomach Cancer Survivors. *Journal of Pain and Symptom Management*, *46*, 511–522. doi:10.1016/j.jpainsymman.2012.10.234

Harris, P. J. & Ferguson, L. R. (1999). Dietary fibres may protect or enhance carcinogenesis. *Mutat. Res.*, *443*, 95–110.

HCN, (2006). Guideline for dietary fibre intake. The Hague, publication n° 2006/03E. Health Council of the Netherlands, Netherlands.

Hernández, A., Martínez, C. & Hernández, M. T. (1995). Fibra alimentaria: Concepto, propiedades y métodos de análisis. Alimentaria: *Revista de tecnología e higiene de los alimentos*, 19–30.

Hillemeier, C. (1995). An overview of the effects of dietary fiber on gastrointestinal transit. *Pediatrics*, *96*, 997–999.

Ho, E., Atwood, J. R., Benedict, J., Ritenbaugh, C., Sheehan, E. T., Abrams, C., Alberts, D. & Meyskens Jr., F.L. (1991). A community-based feasibility study using wheat bran fiber supplementation to lower colon cancer risk. *Preventive Medicine*, *20*, 213–225. doi:10.1016/0091-7435(91)90021-U

Hong, Y., Zi-Jun, W., Jian, X., Ying-jie, D. & Fang, M. (2012). Development of the dietary fiber functional food and studies on its toxicological and physiologic properties. *Food Chem. Toxicol.*, *50*, 3367–3374. doi:10.1016/j.fct.2012.05.011

Howe, G. R., Benito, E., Castelleto, R., Cornée, J., Estève, J., Gallagher, R. P., Iscovich, J. M., Deng-ao, J., Kaaks, R. & Kune, G. A. (1992). Dietary intake of fiber and decreased risk of cancers of the colon and rectum: evidence from the combined analysis of 13 case-control studies. *J. Natl. Cancer Inst.*, *84*, 1887–1896.

IM, (2002). Dietary Reference Intakes for Energy, Carbohydrate, Fiber, Fat, Fatty Acids, Cholesterol, Protein, and Amino Acids (Macronutrients). *Institute of Medicine,* Washington DC.

Jessri, M., Rashidkhani, B., Hajizadeh, B., Jessri, M. & Gotay, C. (2011). Macronutrients, vitamins and minerals intake and risk of esophageal squamous cell carcinoma: a case-control study in Iran. *Nutrition Journal*, *10*, 137. doi:10.1186/1475-2891-10-137

Jiménez-Escrig, A., Rincón, M., Pulido, R. & Saura-Calixto, F. (2001). Guava Fruit (Psidium guajava L.) as a New Source of Antioxidant Dietary Fiber. *J. Agric. Food Chem.*, *49*, 5489–5493. doi:10.1021/jf010147p

Jowett, S. L., Seal, C. J., Phillips, E., Gregory, W., Barton, J. R. & Welfare, M. R. (2004). Dietary beliefs of people with ulcerative colitis and their effect on relapse and nutrient intake. *Clinical Nutrition*, *23*, 161–170. doi:10.1016/S0261-5614(03)00132-8

Kalant, H., Grant, D. & Mitchell, J. (2006). Principles of Medical Pharmacology, 7 edition. ed. Saunders Canada, Toronto, ON.

Kaplan, G. G. (2013). Does Consuming the Recommend Daily Level of Fiber Prevent Crohn's Disease? *Gastroenterology*, *145*, 925–927. doi:10.1053/j.gastro.2013.09.033

Kendall, C. W. C., Esfahani, A. & Jenkins, D. J. A. (2010). The link between dietary fibre and human health. *Food Hydrocolloids*, *24*, 42–48. doi:10.1016/j.foodhyd.2009.08.002.

Khalid, S. A., Musa, A. M., Saeed, A. M., Abugroun, E. A., Sid Ahmed, E. O., Ghalib, M. B., Elnima, E. I., Alkarib, S. Y., Abdelsalam, T. M., Abdelgader, A., Phillips, G. O. & Phillips, A. O. (2014). Manipulating dietary fibre: Gum Arabic making friends of the colon and the kidney. *Bioactive Carbohydrates and Dietary Fibre*, *3*, 71–76. doi:10.1016/j.bcdf.2014.01.005

Khoshoo, V., Sun, S. S. & Storm, H. (2010). Tolerance of an Enteral Formula with Insoluble and Prebiotic Fiber in Children with Compromised Gastrointestinal Function. *Journal of the American Dietetic Association*, *110*, 1728–1733. doi:10.1016/j.jada.2010.08.011

Lewis, S. J. & Heaton, K. W. (1997). The intestinal effects of bran-like plastic particles: is the concept of "roughage" valid after all? *Eur J Gastroenterol Hepatol*, *9*, 553–557.

Lewis, S. J. & Heaton, K. W. (1999). Roughage Revisited (The Effect on Intestinal Function of Inert Plastic Particles of Different Sizes and Shape). *Dig Dis Sci*, *44*, 744–748. doi:10.1023/A:1026613909403

Lochs, H., Steinhardt, H. J., Klaus-Wentz, B., Zeitz, M., Vogelsang, H., Sommer, H., Fleig, W. E., Bauer, P., Schirrmeister, J. & Malchow, H. (1991). Comparison of enteral nutrition and drug treatment in active Crohn's disease. Results of the European Cooperative Crohn's Disease Study. IV. *Gastroenterology*, *101*, 881–888.

Loftus, E. V. (2004). Clinical epidemiology of inflammatory bowel disease: Incidence, prevalence, and environmental influences. *Gastroenterology*, *126*, 1504–1517.

Ludwig, D. S., Pereira, M. A., Kroenke, C. H., Hilner, J. E., Horn, L. V., Slattery, M. L. & Jacobs, D. R. (1999). DIetary fiber, weight gain, and cardiovascular disease risk factors in young adults. *JAMA*, *282*, 1539–1546. doi:10.1001/jama.282.16.1539

Ma, L., Qin, C., Wang, M., Gan, D., Cao, L., Ye, H. & Zeng, X. (2013). Preparation, preliminary characterization and inhibitory effect on human colon cancer HT-29 cells of an acidic polysaccharide fraction from Stachys floridana Schuttl. ex Benth. *Food and Chemical Toxicology*, *60*, 269–276. doi:10.1016/j.fct.2013.07.060

Mann, J. I. & Cummings, J. H. (2009). Possible implications for health of the different definitions of dietary fibre. *Nutr Metab Cardiovasc Dis*, *19*, 226–229. doi:10.1016/j.numecd.2009.02.002

Marlett, J. A., McBurney, M. I., Slavin, J. L. & American Dietetic Association, (2002). Position of the American Dietetic Association: health implications of dietary fiber. *J Am Diet Assoc*, *102*, 993–1000.

Martinho, C., Correia, A., Goncalves, F., Abrantes, J., Carvalho, R. & Guine, R. (2013). Study About the Knowledge and Attitudes of the Portuguese Population About Food Fibres. *Current Nutrition & Food Science*, *9*, 180–188. doi:10.2174/1573401311309030002

McIntosh, G. H., Noakes, M., Royle, P. J. & Foster, P. R. (2003). Whole-grain rye and wheat foods and markers of bowel health in overweight middle-aged men. *Am. J. Clin. Nutr.*, *77*, 967–974.

Møller, M. E., Dahl, R. & Bøckman, O. C. (1988). A possible role of the dietary fibre product, wheat bran, as a nitrite scavenger. *Food Chem. Toxicol.*, *26*, 841–845.

Nakao, M., Ogura, Y., Satake, S., Ito, I., Iguchi, A., Takagi, K. & Nabeshima, T. (2002). Usefulness of soluble dietary fiber for the treatment of diarrhea during enteral nutrition in elderly patients. *Nutrition*, *18*, 35–39. doi:10.1016/S0899-9007(01)00715-8

Navarro Silvera, S. A., Mayne, S. T., Gammon, M. D., Vaughan, T. L., Chow, W. H., Dubin, J. A., Dubrow, R., Stanford, J. L., West, A. B., Rotterdam, H., Blot, W. J. & Risch, H. A. (2014). Diet and lifestyle factors and risk of subtypes of esophageal and gastric cancers: classification tree analysis. *Annals of Epidemiology*, *24*, 50–57. doi:10.1016/j.annepidem.2013.10.009

Nayga, R. J. (1996). Dietary fiber intake away-from-home and at-home in the United States. *Food Policy*, *21*, 279–290.

O'Morain, C., Segal, A. W. & Levi, A. J. (1984). Elemental diet as primary treatment of acute Crohn's disease: a controlled trial. *Br Med J* (Clin Res Ed), *288*, 1859–1862.

O'Neil, C. E., Zanovec, M., Cho, S. S. & Nicklas, T. A. (2010). Whole grain and fiber consumption are associated with lower body weight measures in US adults: National

Health and Nutrition Examination Survey 1999-2004. *Nutr Res*, *30*, 815–822. doi:10.1016/j.nutres.2010.10.013

Occhipinti, K. & Smith, J. W. (2012). Irritable Bowel Syndrome: A Review and Update. *Clin Colon Rectal Surg*, *25*, 46–52. doi:10.1055/s-0032-1301759

Painter, N. S. & Burkitt, D. P. (1971). Diverticular disease of the colon: a deficiency disease of Western civilization. *Br Med J*, *2*, 450–454.

Park, E. J. & Jhon, D. Y. (2009). Effects of bamboo shoot consumption on lipid profiles and bowel function in healthy young women. *Nutrition*, *25*, 723–728. doi:10.1016/j.nut.2009.01.007

Park, Y., Brinton, L. A., Subar, A. F., Hollenbeck, A. & Schatzkin, A. (2009). Dietary fiber intake and risk of breast cancer in postmenopausal women: the National Institutes of Health-AARP Diet and Health Study. *Am. J. Clin. Nutr.*, *90*, 664–671. doi:10.3945/ajcn.2009.27758

Reddy, B. S. (1999). Role of dietary fiber in colon cancer: an overview. The American *Journal of Medicine*, *106*, 16–19. doi:10.1016/S0002-9343(98)00341-6

Reddy, B. S. & Mori, H. (1981). Effect of dietary wheat bran and dehydrated citrus fiber on 3,2'-dimethyl-4-aminobiphenyl-induced intestinal carcinogenesis in F344 rats. *Carcinogenesis*, *2*, 21–25.

Reddy, B. S., Mori, H. & Nicolais, M. (1981). Effect of dietary wheat bran and dehydrated citrus fiber on azoxymethane-induced intestinal carcinogenesis in Fischer 344 rats. *J. Natl. Cancer Inst.*, *66*, 553–557.

Rodríguez, R., Jiménez, A., Fernández-Bolaños, J., Guillén, R. & Heredia, A. (2006). Dietary fibre from vegetable products as source of functional ingredients. *Trends in Food Science & Technology*, *17*, 3–15. doi:10.1016/j.tifs.2005.10.002

Rosamond, W. D. (2002). Dietary fiber and prevention of cardiovascular disease**. *J Am Coll Cardiol*, *39*, 57–59. doi:10.1016/S0735-1097(01)01685-0

Rushdi, T. A., Pichard, C. & Khater, Y. H. (2004). Control of diarrhea by fiber-enriched diet in ICU patients on enteral nutrition: a prospective randomized controlled trial. *Clinical Nutrition*, *23*, 1344–1352. doi:10.1016/j.clnu.2004.04.008

Russel, M. G., Engels, L. G., Muris, J. W., Limonard, C. B., Volovics, A., Brummer, R. J. & Stockbrügger, R. W. (1998). Modern life' in the epidemiology of inflammatory bowel disease: a case-control study with special emphasis on nutritional factors. *Eur J Gastroenterol Hepatol*, *10*, 243–249.

Saldanha, H. (1999). Nutrição Clínica. Lidel, Lisbon, Portugal.

Sardinha, A. N., Canella, D. S., Martins, A. P. B., Claro, R. M. & Levy, R. B. (2014). Dietary sources of fiber intake in Brazil. *Appetite*, 79, 134–138. doi:10.1016/j.appet.2014.04.018

Scharlau, D., Borowicki, A., Habermann, N., Hofmann, T., Klenow, S., Miene, C., Munjal, U., Stein, K. & Glei, M. (2009). Mechanisms of primary cancer prevention by butyrate and other products formed during gut flora-mediated fermentation of dietary fibre. *Mutation Research/Reviews in Mutation Research*, *682*, 39–53. doi:10.1016/j.mrrev.2009.04.001

Schatzkin, A., Park, Y., Leitzmann, M. F., Hollenbeck, A. R. & Cross, A. J. (2008). Prospective study of dietary fiber, whole grain foods, and small intestinal cancer. *Gastroenterology*, *135*, 1163–1167. doi:10.1053/j.gastro.2008.07.015

Seidner, D. L., Lashner, B. A., Brzezinski, A., Banks, P. L. C., Goldblum, J., Fiocchi, C., Katz, J., Lichtenstein, G. R., Anton, P. A., Kam, L. Y., Garleb, K. A. & Demichele, S. J.

(2005). An oral supplement enriched with fish oil, soluble fiber, and antioxidants for corticosteroid sparing in ulcerative colitis: A randomized, controlled trial. *Clinical Gastroenterology and Hepatology*, *3*, 358–369. doi:10.1016/S1542-3565(04)00672-X

Sjöberg, D., Holmström, T., Larsson, M., Nielsen, A. L., Holmquist, L., Ekbom, A. & Rönnblom, A. (2014). Incidence and clinical course of Crohn's disease during the first year — Results from the IBD Cohort of the Uppsala Region (ICURE) of Sweden 2005–2009. *Journal of Crohn's and Colitis*, *8*, 215–222. doi:10.1016/j.crohns.2013.08.009

Slavin, J. L. (2003). Impact of the proposed definition of dietary fiber on nutrient databases. Journal of Food Composition and Analysis, 26th *International Nutrient Database Conference*, *16*, 287–291. doi:10.1016/S0889-1575(03)00053-X

Slavin, J. L. (2005). Dietary fiber and body weight. *Nutrition*, *21*, 411–418. doi:10.1016/j.nut.2004.08.018

Slavin, J. L. (2008). Position of the American Dietetic Association: health implications of dietary fiber. *J Am Diet Assoc*, *108*, 1716–1731.

Stange, E. F., Travis, S. P. L., Vermeire, S., Beglinger, C., Kupcinskas, L., Geboes, K., Barakauskiene, A., Villanacci, V., Von Herbay, A., Warren, B.F., Gasche, C., Tilg, H., Schreiber, S. W., Scholmerich, J. & Reinisch, W. (2006). European evidence based consensus on the diagnosis and management of Crohn's disease: definitions and diagnosis. *Gut*, *55*, i1–i15. doi:10.1136/gut.2005.081950a

Stefanelli, T., Malesci, A., Repici, A., Vetrano, S. & Danese, S. (2008). New insights into inflammatory bowel disease pathophysiology: paving the way for novel therapeutic targets. *Curr Drug Targets*, *9*, 413–418.

Stein, A. C. & Cohen, R. D. (2014). Dietary Fiber Intake and Crohn's Disease. *Gastroenterology*, *146*, 1133. doi:10.1053/j.gastro.2013.12.044

Stein, K., Borowicki, A., Scharlau, D., Schettler, A., Scheu, K., Obst, U. & Glei, M. (2012). Effects of synbiotic fermentation products on primary chemoprevention in human colon cells. *The Journal of Nutritional Biochemistry*, *23*, 777–784. doi:10.1016/j.jnutbio.2011.03.022

Stollman, N. & Raskin, J. B. (2004). Diverticular disease of the colon. *The Lancet*, *363*, 631–639. doi:10.1016/S0140-6736(04)15597-9

Suwannaporn, P., Thepwong, K., Tester, R., Al-Ghazzewi, F., Piggott, J., Shen, N., Chen, Z., Chen, F., Yang, J., Zhang, D. & Tang, M. (2013). Tolerance and nutritional therapy of dietary fibre from konjac glucomannan hydrolysates for patients with inflammatory bowel disease (IBD). *Bioactive Carbohydrates and Dietary Fibre*, *2*, 93–98. doi:10.1016/j.bcdf.2013.09.005

Tang, L., Xu, F., Zhang, T., Lei, J., Binns, C. W. & Lee, A. H. (2013). Dietary fibre intake associated with reduced risk of oesophageal cancer in Xinjiang, China. *Cancer Epidemiology*, *37*, 893–896. doi:10.1016/j.canep.2013.08.012

Teahon, K., Smethurst, P., Pearson, M., Levi, A. J. & Bjarnason, I. (1991). The effect of elemental diet on intestinal permeability and inflammation in Crohn's disease. *Gastroenterology*, *101*, 84–89.

Terry, P., Lagergren, J., Ye, W., Wolk, A. & Nyrén, O. (2001). Inverse association between intake of cereal fiber and risk of gastric cardia cancer. *Gastroenterology*, *120*, 387–391.

Thompson, W. G. (2000). Constipation: a physiological approach. *Can. J. Gastroenterol.*, *14,* Suppl D, 155D–162D.

Thrift, A. P., Pandeya, N. & Whiteman, D. C. (2012). Current status and future perspectives on the etiology of esophageal adenocarcinoma. *Front Oncol*, *2*, 11. doi:10.3389/fonc.2012.00011.

Tramonte, S. M., Brand, M. B., Mulrow, C. D., Amato, M. G., O'Keefe, M. E. & Ramirez, G. (1997). The treatment of chronic constipation in adults. A systematic review. *J Gen Intern Med*, *12*, 15–24.

Trock, B., Lanza, E. & Greenwald, P. (1990). Dietary fiber, vegetables, and colon cancer: critical review and meta-analyses of the epidemiologic evidence. *J. Natl. Cancer Inst.*, *82*, 650–661.

Tudoran, A., Olsen, S. O. & Dopico, D. C. (2009). The effect of health benefit information on consumers health value, attitudes and intentions. *Appetite*, *52*, 568–579. doi:10.1016/j.appet.2009.01.009

Van Duyn, M. A. S. & Pivonka, E. (2000). Overview of the Health Benefits of Fruit and Vegetable Consumption for the Dietetics Professional: Selected Literature. *Journal of the American Dietetic Association*, *100*, 1511–1521. doi:10.1016/S0002-8223(00)00420-X

Van Loo, E. S., Dijkstra, G., Ploeg, R. J. & Nieuwenhuijs, V. B. (2012). Prevention of postoperative recurrence of Crohn's disease. *Journal of Crohn's and Colitis*, *6*, 637–646. doi:10.1016/j.crohns.2011.12.006

Van Loo, J., Cummings, J., Delzenne, N., Englyst, H., Franck, A., Hopkins, M., Kok, N., Macfarlane, G., Newton, D., Quigley, M., Roberfroid, M., van Vliet, T. & van den Heuvel, E. (1999). Functional food properties of non-digestible oligosaccharides: a consensus report from the ENDO project (DGXII AIRII-CT94-1095). *Br. J. Nutr.*, *81*, 121–132.

Vincent, R., Roberts, A., Frier, M., Perkins, A. C., MacDonald, I. A. & Spiller, R. C. (1995). Effect of bran particle size on gastric emptying and small bowel transit in humans: a scintigraphic study. *Gut*, *37*, 216–219.

Wald, A. (2007). Chronic constipation: advances in management. *Neurogastroenterol. Motil.*, *19*, 4–10. doi:10.1111/j.1365-2982.2006.00835.x

Wanders, A. J., van den Borne, J. J. G. C., de Graaf, C., Hulshof, T., Jonathan, M. C., Kristensen, M., Mars, M., Schols, H. A. & Feskens, E. J. M. (2011). Effects of dietary fibre on subjective appetite, energy intake and body weight: a systematic review of randomized controlled trials. *Obes Rev*, *12*, 724–739. doi:10.1111/j.1467-789X.2011.00895.x

Wasan, H. S. & Goodlad, R. A. (1996). Fibre-supplemented foods may damage your health. *Lancet*, *348*, 319–320.

Wess, L., Eastwood, M. A., Edwards, C. A., Busuttil, A., Miller, A. (1996). Collagen alteration in an animal model of colonic diverticulosis. *Gut*, *38*, 701–706.

Wu, A. H., Tseng, C. C., Hankin, J. & Bernstein, L. (2007). Fiber intake and risk of adenocarcinomas of the esophagus and stomach. *Cancer Causes Control*, *18*, 713–722. doi:10.1007/s10552-007-9014-8

Yen, C. H., Tseng, Y. H., Kuo, Y. W., Lee, M. C. & Chen, H. L. (2011). Long-term supplementation of isomalto-oligosaccharides improved colonic microflora profile, bowel function, and blood cholesterol levels in constipated elderly people—A placebo-controlled, diet-controlled trial. *Nutrition*, *27*, 445–450. doi:10.1016/j.nut.2010.05.012

Zhang, N., Huang, C. & Ou, S. (2011). In vitro binding capacities of three dietary fibers and their mixture for four toxic elements, cholesterol, and bile acid. *J. Hazard. Mater.*, *186*, 236–239. doi:10.1016/j.jhazmat.2010.10.120

Zhang, Z., Xu, G., Ma, M., Yang, J. & Liu, X. (2013). Dietary Fiber Intake Reduces Risk for Gastric Cancer: A Meta-analysis. *Gastroenterology*, *145*, 113–120.e3. doi:10.1053/j.gastro.2013.04.001

In: Dietary Fiber
Editor: Marvin E. Clemens

ISBN: 978-1-63463-655-1
© 2015 Nova Science Publishers, Inc.

Chapter 3

LONG EXPOSURE TO THE PREBIOTICS NUTRIOSE® FB06 AND RAFTILOSE® P95 INCREASES UPTAKE OF THE SHORT-CHAIN FATTY ACID BUTYRATE BY INTESTINAL EPITHELIAL CELLS

Cátia Costa[1], Pedro Gonçalves[1,2], Ana Correia-Branco[1] and Fátima Martel[1,*]

[1]Department of Biochemistry (U38-FCT), Faculty of Medicine of Porto, University of Porto, Portugal

[2]Institut Necker Enfants Malades (INEM)/Medical Faculty Descartes, Paris, France

ABSTRACT

We aimed to evaluate the effect of the prebiotics Nutriose® FB06 (NUT) and Raftilose® P95 (RAF) upon uptake of ^{14}C-butyrate (^{14}C-BT), and upon its cellular effects, in a rat normal intestinal epithelial cell line (IEC-6 cells). A long exposure (48h) to NUT or RAF (20-100 mg/ml) caused an increase in ^{14}C-BT uptake. This effect involved the sodium-dependent monocarboxylate transporter 1 (SMCT1) but not the proton-coupled monocarboxylate 1 transporter (MCT1), although prebiotics showed no effect on SMCT1 and MCT1 mRNA expression levels. BT (5 mM; 48h) markedly decreased cellular viability and culture growth and increased cell differentiation. Combination of prebiotics with BT did not significantly modify these parameters. In conclusion, the results show that a long exposure to NUT and RAF increases uptake of a low concentration of ^{14}C-BT by intestinal epithelial cells, although the prebiotics do not modify the effects of BT upon cell viability, culture growth and differentiation.

Keywords: Prebiotics, butyrate, cellular uptake, sodium-dependent monocarboxylate transporter 1, anticarcinogenic effect

* Corresponding author: F. Martel. Department of Biochemistry, Faculty of Medicine of Porto, 4200-319 Porto, Portugal. Phone: 351 22 0426654. Fax: 351 22 5513624. Email: fmartel@med.up.pt.

INTRODUCTION

Inflammatory bowel disease (IBD) are chronic inflammatory disorders of the gastrointestinal tract that affect more than 3 million people worldwide (Loftus, 2004) and colorectal cancer (CRC) is a very common malignancy and a prime cause of cancer death in developed countries (Jemal et al., 2010). Dietary fiber is one of the most promising candidates for a protective role in IBD (Jakobsen et al., 2013) and CRC development (Young et al., 2005). One of the mechanisms by which dietary fiber promotes colonic health is through its fermentation by gut microbiota (*Bacteroidetes* and *Firmicutes*) resulting in the production of short-chain fatty acids (SCFA) (Topping and Clifton, 2001). Therefore, SCFA have been suggested to be the link between dietary fiber, microbiota and colon homeostasis (Ganapathy et al., 2013). Butyrate (BT) is a SCFA known to play a key role in colonic epithelium homeostasis. Its beneficial effects on the prevention/inhibition of colon inflammation and carcinogenesis (Hamer et al., 2008; Canani et al., 2011) are mediated at least partly by its ability to inhibit histone deacetylases (Davie, 2004), which is dependent on a previous uptake by colonocytes. BT is taken up into colonic epithelial cells by two specific carrier-mediated transport systems: the proton-coupled monocarboxylate transporter 1 (MCT1) and the sodium-coupled monocarboxylate transporter 1 (SMCT1). In agreement with the fact that the anticarcinogenic effects of BT are dependent on its cellular uptake, both MCT1 and SMCT1 were proposed to function as tumor suppressors (Cuff et al., 2005; Gupta et al., 2006).

The well-recognized health benefits of dietary fiber (Ganapathy et al., 2013) provides the basis for the promotion of the use of prebiotics in current clinical practice (Balakrishnan and Floch, 2012; Quigley, 2012). Prebiotics are defined as nondigestible food ingredients (complex carbohydrates) that can be fermented by colonic bacteria and that beneficially affect the host by selectively stimulating the growth or the activity of one or a limited number of bacteria (eg. bifidobacteria, lactobacilli) in the colon (Gibson et al., 2004). Nutriose® FB 06 (NUT) is a commercially available prebiotic produced from wheat starch, with up to 85% of fiber content (dry substance). It consists of a mixture of glucose polymers with a high number of α-1,6 linkages and non-digestible glucoside linkages such as α-1,2 and α-1,3, with a narrow range of molecular weight and a degree of polymerization (DP) range of 12 to 15 (Lefranc-Millot, 2008). It has been shown to be mostly resistant to digestion in the small intestine (15% is enzymatically digested, 75% is slowly and progressively fermented in the colon, SCFA, and 10% is excreted) (van den Heuvel et al., 2004). The prebiotic Raftilose® P95 (RAF), a commercially available oligofructose, is obtained from enzyme hydrolysis of chicory inulin. It is composed of a mixture of glucosyl-(fructosyl)n-fructose (64%) and (fructosyl)n-fructose (36%) and has a DP range of 2 to 8. Unlike NUT, RAF reaches the colon practically intact, where it is fermented, leading to the production of SCFA (Niness, 1999).

Interestingly, in a recent report, the serum concentrations of acetate and propionate were increased in rats fed standard diet supplemented with the prebiotics NUT or RAF but, unexpectedly, the serum concentrations of BT were unchanged or even decreased (Kosmus et al., 2011). Because nothing was known concerning the putative influence of prebiotics on the cellular uptake of BT, we hypothesized that these prebiotics could interfere with the colonic epithelial uptake of BT. Therefore, we decided to investigate the influence of the prebiotics NUT and RAF on the cellular uptake of BT by normal intestinal epithelial cells.

METHODS AND MATERIALS

IEC-6 Cell Culture

The IEC-6 cell line was obtained from Deutsche Sammlung von Mikroorganismen und Zellkulturen (ACC-111; Braunschweig, Germany) and used between passages 17 and 28. The cells were maintained in a humidified atmosphere of 5% CO_2–95% air and cultured in Dulbecco's modified Eagle medium:RPMI 1640 medium (1:1) (Sigma, St. Louis, MO) supplemented with 10% fetal bovine serum (Invitrogen Corp., Carlsbad, CA), 0.1 U/ml insulin, 5.96 g HEPES, 2.2 g $NaHCO_3$, 100 units/ml penicillin, 100 µg/ml streptomycin and 0.25 µg/ml amphotericin B (all from Sigma). Culture medium was changed every 2–3 days, and the culture was split every 7 days. For subculturing, cells were removed enzymatically (0.05% trypsin-EDTA, 5 min, 37°C), split 1:3 and subcultured in plastic culture dishes (21 cm^2; ∅ 60 mm; Corning Costar, Corning, NY). For use in experiments, IEC-6 cells were seeded on 24-well plastic cell culture clusters (2 cm^2; ∅ 16 mm, Corning Costar) (uptake, cytotoxicity, culture growth and cell differentiation assays) or on plastic culture dishes (21 cm^2; ∅ 60 mm; Corning Costar) (qRT-PCR). The experiments were performed 7-9 days after the initial seeding (90–100% confluence). For 24 h before the experiments, the cell medium was made free of fetal calf serum and insulin.

Treatment of the Cells

The acute effect of the prebiotics was tested by incubating cells in glucose-free Krebs (GFK) buffer (containing, in mM: 125 NaCl, 25 $NaHCO_3$, 4.8 KCl, 0.4 K_2HPO_4, 1.6 KH_2PO_4, 1.2 $MgSO_4$, 1.2 $CaCl_2$ and 20 MES (pH 6.5)) for 1, 3 or 6h in the presence of these compounds (1, 5, 10, 20, 50 or 100 mg/ml) or the isosmolar concentration of manitol.

The chronic effect of prebiotics and/or butyrate was tested by cultivating cell cultures at 6–8 days of age (90–95% confluence) in culture medium in the presence of the compounds to be tested. The medium was renewed daily, and the experiments were performed after 48 h.

Determination of ^{14}C-BT Uptake

Uptake experiments were performed with cells incubated in GFK buffer (pH 6.5). Initially, the culture medium was aspirated and the cells were washed with 0.3 ml buffer at 37°C. Then, cells were incubated with GFK medium at 37°C containing ^{14}C-BT (10 µM) for 3 min. Afterwards, incubation was stopped by removing the buffer, placing the cells on ice and rinsing the cells with 0.3 ml ice-cold GFK buffer. Cells were then solubilized with 0.3 ml 0.1% (v/v) Triton X-100 (in 5 mM Tris-HCl, pH 7.4) and placed at 37°C overnight. Radioactivity in the cells was measured by liquid scintillation counting.

In some experiments, the sodium-dependence (by using GFK buffer in which NaCl was isotonically substituted with LiCl) and the effect of inhibitors (NPPB and pCMB) were tested by preincubating (for 20 min) and then incubating cells with ^{14}C-BT (for 3 min) in the absence or presence of these conditions.

Protein Determination

The protein content of cell monolayers was determined as described by Bradford (1976), using human serum albumin as standard.

Evaluation of Cell Viability (Quantification of Extracellular Lactate Dehydrogenase (LDH) Activity)

After treatment, cellular leakage of the cytosolic enzyme LDH into the extracellular medium was measured spectrophotometrically by measuring the decrease in absorbance of NADH during the reduction of pyruvate to lactate, as described previously (Gonçalves et al., 2011a; Gonçalves et al., 2012). The amount of LDH present in the extracellular medium, which correlates with cell death, was then calculated as a percentage of the total LDH activity.

Evaluation of Culture Growth (Sulforhodamine B (SRB) Assay)

After treatment, quantification of the whole-cell protein with the SRB assay was performed as described elsewhere (Gonçalves et al., 2011a; Gonçalves et al., 2012).

Determination of Cellular Differentiation (Alkaline Phosphatase (ALP) Activity Assay)

After the treatment period, cell differentiation was measured by quantification of ALP activity, as previously described (Gonçalves et al., 2012). ALP activity was determined spectrophotometrically by using p-nitrophenylphosphate as substrate, and the results were expressed as nmol p-nitrophenol$\cdot$min$^{-1}\cdot$mg protein^{-1}.

Real-Time Quantitative Reverse Transcription Polymerase Chain Reaction (qRT-PCR)

Extraction of total RNA and qRT-PCR were carried out as described recently by our group (Gonçalves et al., 2013).

Calculations and Statistics

Arithmetic means are given with SEM. Statistical significance of the difference between two groups was evaluated by one-tailed Student's t-test; statistical analysis of the difference between various groups was evaluated by the analysis of variance test, followed by the Student-Newman-Keuls test. Differences were considered to be significant when a P value of less than 0.05.

MATERIALS

[^{14}C]BT ([1-^{14}C]-n-butyric acid, sodium salt; specific activity 30–60 mCi/mmol) (Biotrend Chemikalien GmbH, Koln, Germany); NUT (Roquette Frères, Lestrem, France); RAF (Raffinerie Tirlemontoise, Tienen, Belgium); acetic acid, ethanol, manitol, MES ((2-[N-morpholino] ethanesulfonic acid hydrate)), NADH (nicotinamide adenine dinucleotide), NaOH, p-nitrophenylphosphate, NPPB (5-nitro-2-(3-phenylpropylamino)benzoic acid), pCMB (4-(hydroxymercuri)benzoic acid sodium salt), RNAseOUT™, serum albumin, sodium butyrate, sodium pyruvate, sulforhodamine B, Superscript Reverse transcriptase II, trichloroacetic acid sodium salt, Tris–HCl, Tris.NaOH, trypsin–EDTA solution (Sigma, St. Louis, MO, USA); triton X-100 (Merck, Darmstadt, Germany); LightCycler FastStart DNA MasterPlus SYBR Green I, Tripure® kit (Roche Diagnostics, Germany); DNAse I, RNAse H (Invitrogen Corp. Carlsbad, CA, USA).

Compounds to be tested were dissolved in H_2O or dimethylsulfoxide. The final concentration of these solvents in the buffer was 1%. Controls for these compounds were run in the presence of the respective solvent.

RESULTS

Short-Exposure to Prebiotics

In a first series of experiments, we evaluated the effect of a short exposure (3h) to NUT and RAF (1-20 mg/ml) upon ^{14}C-BT uptake. As shown in Figure 1, apart from an inhibitory effect found with NUT (20 mg/ml), no significant effect was found. The inhibitory effect of NUT was not related with a cytotoxic or inhibitory effect on culture growth (results not shown). When tested in higher concentrations (50 and 100 mg/ml) and over a time range (1-6h), neither of the prebiotics was able to significantly affect ^{14}C-BT uptake (similarly, these higher concentrations of the compounds did not present a cytotoxic effect; results not shown).

Long-Exposure to Prebiotics

In the second series of experiments, a longer exposure (48h) to NUT and RAF (20-100 mg/ml) was tested. As shown in Figure 2, uptake of ^{14}C-BT by IEC-6 cells was increased by both prebiotics (20-100 mg/ml), by a maximum of about 35-40% (observed with NUT 50 mg/ml and RAF 20 mg/ml). Neither of these concentrations presented a cytotoxic or inhibitory effect upon culture growth (results not shown).

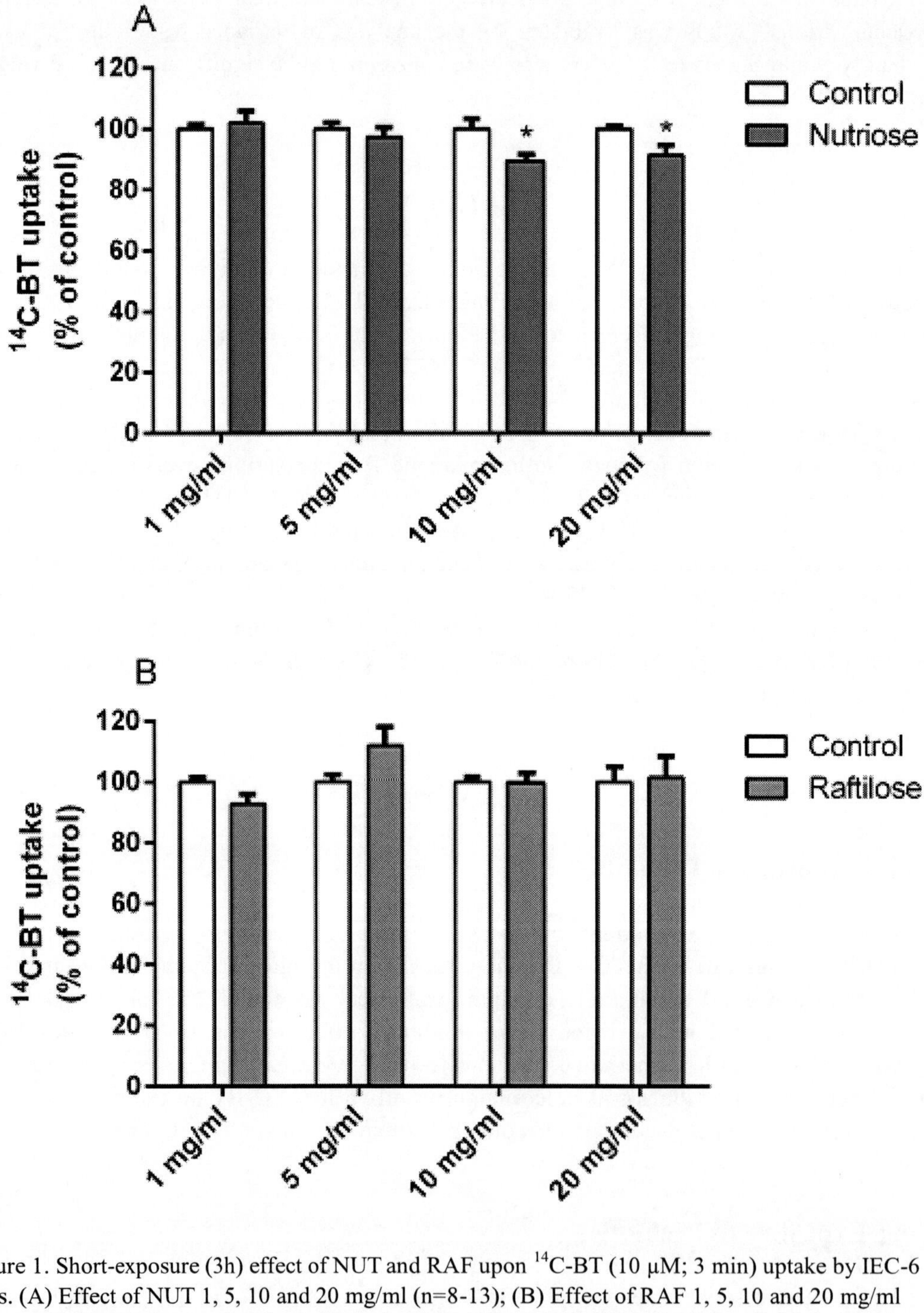

Figure 1. Short-exposure (3h) effect of NUT and RAF upon ^{14}C-BT (10 μM; 3 min) uptake by IEC-6 cells. (A) Effect of NUT 1, 5, 10 and 20 mg/ml (n=8-13); (B) Effect of RAF 1, 5, 10 and 20 mg/ml (n=13-15). Results are presented as arithmetic means±SEM. * Significantly different from control (*P*<0.05) (Student's t test).

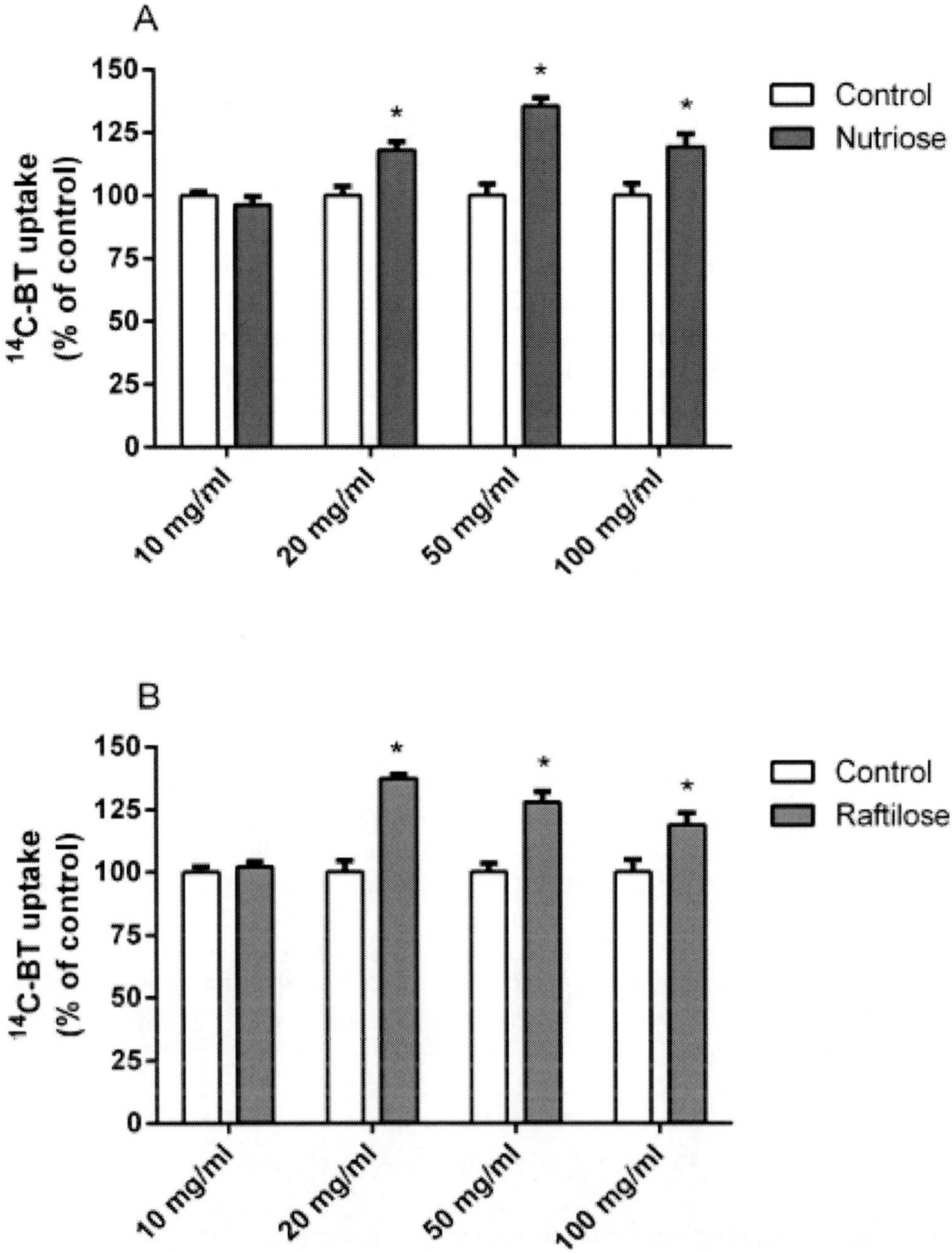

Figure 2. Long-exposure (48h) effect of NUT and RAF upon ^{14}C-BT (10 μM; 3 min) uptake by IEC-6 cells. (A) Effect of NUT 10, 20, 50 and 100 mg/ml (n=8-9); (B) Effect of RAF 10, 20, 50 and 100 mg/ml (n=8-9). Results are presented as arithmetic means±SEM. * Significantly different from control (*P*<0.05) (Student's t test).

In a recent report from our group, uptake of ^{14}C-BT by IEC-6 cells was concluded to involve both MCT1 and SMCT1, based in the presence of both sodium-dependent and independent components of uptake (SMCT1- and MCT1-mediated, respectively) together with the expression of both MCT1 and SMCT1 mRNA by these cells (Gonçalves et al. 2011b). So, we decided to investigate the effect of NUT (50 mg/ml) and RAF (20 mg/ml) upon both components of ^{14}C-BT uptake. In agreement with the previous report, ^{14}C-BT uptake was found to be mainly sodium-independent, although a sodium-dependent component of uptake, corresponding to about 30% of total uptake, was also present (Figure 3). Interestingly, although both NUT and RAF increased total ^{14}C-BT uptake (Figure 2 and Figure 3), they showed no effect on the sodium-independent component of uptake. The conclusion that both prebiotics have no effect upon MCT1-mediated ^{14}C-BT uptake was reinforced when we used specific MCT1 inhibitors (NPPB and pCMB) (Gonçalves et al. 2011b) that allowed us to discriminate the MCT1-mediated component of sodium-independent ^{14}C-BT uptake (Figure 3). So, we conclude that NUT and RAF present a specific stimulatory effect solely upon SMCT1-mediated ^{14}C-BT uptake. However, NUT (50 mg/ml) and RAF (20 mg/ml) (48h) did not affect SMCT1 mRNA expression and they were devoid of effect upon MCT1 mRNA expression as well (results not shown).

BT exerts a potent antiproliferative/anticarcinogenic effect in many intestinal tumoral cell lines (Hamer et al. 2008), and it was also recently found to inhibit cell growth, decrease viability and induce cellular differentiation of IEC-6 cells (Gonçalves et al. 2011a). Because the most important molecular mechanisms involved in the anticarcinogenic effect of BT are dependent on its intracellular concentration (e.g., inhibition of histone deacetylases) (Davie, 2004), in a final series of experiments, we aimed to investigate if the increase in ^{14}C-BT uptake induced by NUT (50 mg/ml) and RAF (20 mg/ml) would change the effects of BT upon cell viability, culture growth and cell differentiation. In agreement with our previous report, BT (5 mM) caused a significant decrease in cellular viability and culture growth and a significant increase in cell differentiation (Figure 4). However, NUT and RAF were not able to cause a significant change in these cellular effects of BT (5 mM). Moreover, we also tested BT 1 mM; this concentration of BT caused a significant decrease in culture growth (to 72.3±16% of control; n=12) but was not able to modify cell viability and differentiation (results not shown). Again, both prebiotics did not modify the effect of BT upon these parameters (results not shown).

Discussion and Conclusion

Prebiotics, by causing significant changes in the composition of the gut microflora (with increased and reduced numbers of potentially health-promoting bacteria and potentially harmful species, respectively), regulate the capacity of bacteria to generate SCFA such as BT (Roberfroid, 2007). Interestingly, gut microbiome analysis has revealed a significant decrease in the number of SCFA and BT-producing bacteria in the colon of IBD and CRC patients (Frank et al., 2007; Sokol et al., 2009; Wang et al., 2012), and the use of prebiotics in current clinical practice in these patients (Balakrishnan and Floch, 2012; Quigley, 2012) probably results in an increased concentration of BT in the colon. However, it also increases the concentration of not fermented prebiotics. So, in vivo, both are present in the colon. In a recent report, in which rats were fed with standard diet supplemented with the prebiotics NUT or RAF, serum concentrations of acetate and propionate were increased, but the serum concentrations of BT were unchanged or even decreased (Kosmus et al., 2011). So, the aim of this study was to investigate the relationship between NUT and RAF and the cellular uptake of BT by intestinal epithelial cells, because we hypothesized that they could interfere with this process.

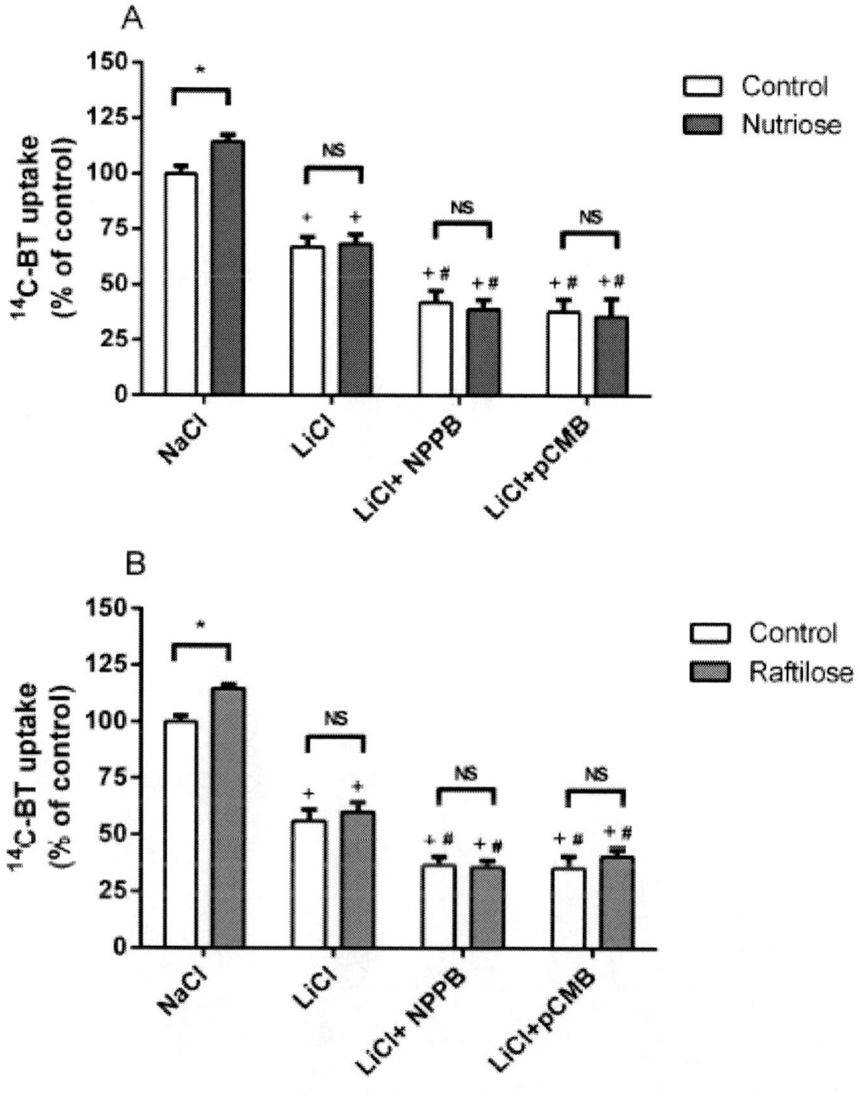

Figure 3. Long-exposure (48h) effect of NUT and RAF upon SMCT1- and MCT1-mediated ^{14}C-BT uptake by IEC-6 cells. Effect of (A) NUT 50 mg/ml (n=9) and (B) RAF 20 mg/ml (n=8-9) on ^{14}C-BT uptake (10 μM; 3 min) in the presence (NaCl) or absence of NaCl in the GFK buffer (LiCl), under control conditions or in the presence of 5-nitro-2-(3-phenylpropylamino)benzoic acid (NPPB) 0.5 mM or p-chloromercuribenzoate (pCMB) 0.5 mM. Results are presented as arithmetic means±SEM. * Significantly different from control (P<0.05; Student's t test); $^{+}$ significantly different from NaCl and $^{\#}$ significantly different from LiCl (P<0.05; ANOVA + Student-Newman-Keuls test).

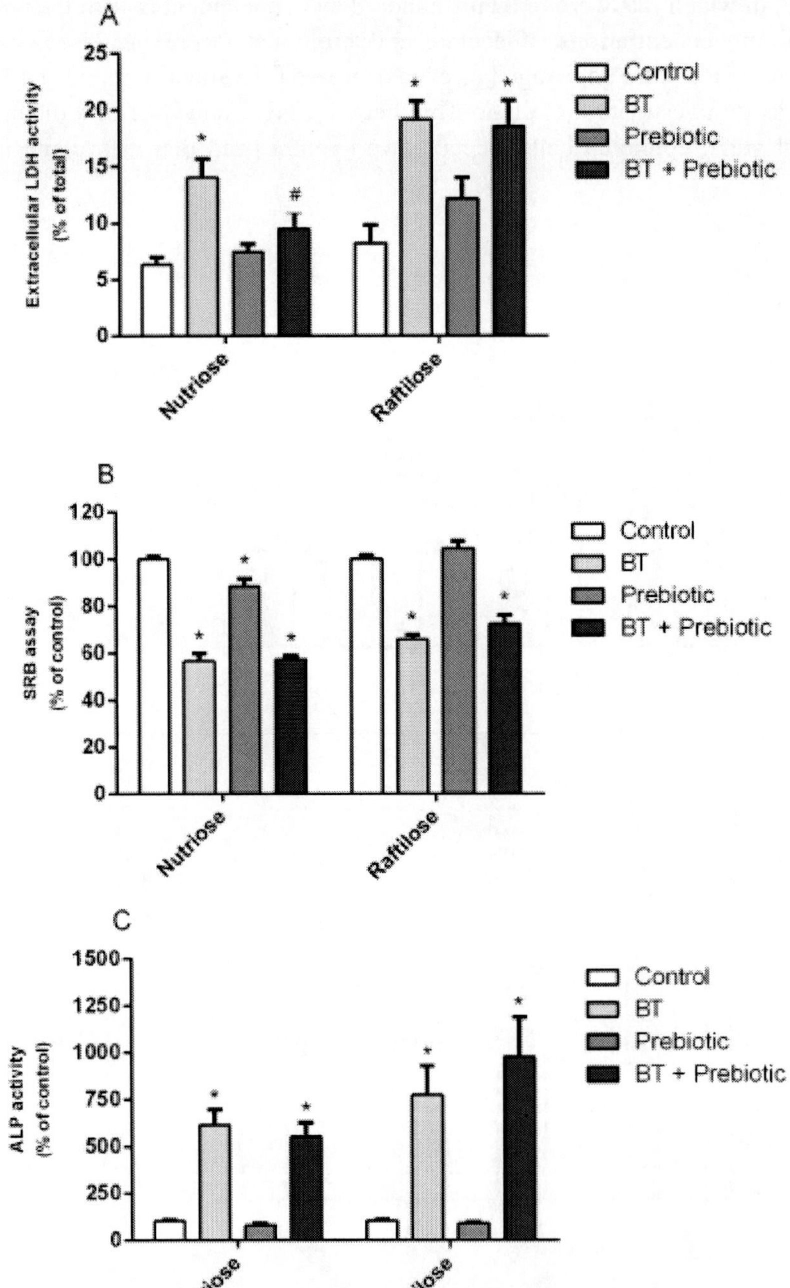

Figure 4. Effect of a 48h-exposure to BT (5 mM), NUT (50 mg/ml), RAF (20 mg/ml) or a combination of both compounds (BT + NUT or BT + RAF) on (A) cell viability, determined by quantification of extracellular LDH activity (n=21-24); (B) culture growth, determined by quantification of whole cell protein with SRB (n=10-12); and (C) cell differentiation, determined by quantification of ALP activity (n=15-17). * Significantly different from control (P<0.05); # significantly different from BT (5 mM) (P<0.05 ; ANOVA + Student-Newman-Keuls test).

We verified that a long-term exposure of IEC-6 cells to the prebiotics NUT and RAF increased total BT cellular uptake, mediated by a specific stimulatory effect upon SMCT1 and independent of changes in SMCT1 transcription rates. To our knowledge, this is the first report on the effect of prebiotics on BT transport activity and BT transporter expression levels. MCT1 was recently found to be upregulated along the gastrointestinal tract of pectin-fed rats. This was discussed by the authors as representing an adaptive response to the increased availability of its substrates (Kirat et al., 2009). Indeed, MCT1 is known to be upregulated by BT (Cuff et al., 2002). However, in the present work, a direct *in vitro* effect of the prebiotics is described. So, besides being a primary source of BT, NUT and RAF also appear to increase the uptake of BT by intestinal epithelial cells, thus adding another mechanism to their beneficial effects at colonic level. Other well-recognized beneficial effects of prebiotics are also known to be present. For instance, they have direct in vitro immunomodulatory (Eiwegger et al., 2010), anti-inflammatory (Zehnon et al., 2011) and antiproliferative effects (Asai et al., 2011) and they inhibit the adherence of pathogens (Shoaf et al., 2006).

Because the most important molecular mechanisms involved in the anticarcinogenic effect of BT are dependent on its intracellular concentration (e.g., inhibition of histone deacetylases) (Davie, 2004), we decided to investigate if the prebiotics were able to modify the effects of BT upon cell viability and differentiation and culture growth. However, despite a stimulatory effect exerted by both NUT and RAF on BT cellular uptake, the prebiotics were not able to significantly interfere with these cellular effects of BT. One possible explanation for this observation is that BT elicits uptake-independent biologic antiproliferative/ anticarcinogenic effects on intestinal epithelial cells (eg. GPR109A or GPR43-mediated) (Ganapathy et al., 2013). However, we hypothesize that the lack of effect of prebiotics in modulating these cellular effects of BT may be related to the fact that SMCT1 has a high affinity for BT (the Michaelis constant for BT transport is about 50 μM; Miyauchi et al., 2004). Interestingly, there was no difference in the incidence of colon cancer in SMCT1-null mice under optimal dietary fiber conditions, but under low-fiber dietary conditions, the incidence of colon cancer was much higher (Ganapathy et al., 2013). This clearly suggests that SMCT1 is the most important BT transporter when BT concentrations are low. So, the stimulatory effect of prebiotics upon SMCT1 would be evident upon transport of ^{14}C-BT (which was carried out with a substrate concentration of 10 μM) but would not be seen when a much higher concentration of BT (5 mM) was used. This concentration of BT (5 mM), which is well within the physiological concentration of this SCFA at colonic luminal level (Ganapathy et al., 2013), clearly presents an inhibitory effect upon viability and culture growth and a pro-differentiation effect. At such high concentrations of BT, significant amounts of BT may enter cells via diffusion or via the other monocarboxylate transporter, MCT1, which exhibits a much lower affinity for BT (Gonçalves et al., 2011b). In order to investigate if the stimulatory effect of prebiotics would become apparent at lower concentrations of BT, we tested BT 1 mM. However, it became evident that BT at this concentration was devoid of significant effects upon these cellular parameters. So, we could not further investigate this point. Nevertheless, we hypothesize that these prebiotics may not have noticeable effects on BT cellular effects (eg. tumor supression) when dietary fiber intake is optimal, but they may enhance uptake of BT by colonic epithelial cells, and in such a way have a tumor suppressive effect, under conditions causing colonic low concentrations of BT (eg. absent or low dietary fiber intake or chronic use of antibiotics).

In conclusion, this work shows a stimulatory effect of the prebiotics NUT and RAF upon uptake of low concentrations of BT by intestinal epithelial cells, mediated by a specific effect upon SMCT1 activity and not related to changes in SMCT1 expression levels.

Abbreviations

BT	butyrate
NUT	Nutriose® FB06
RAF	Raftilose® P95
SCFA	short-chain fatty acids

Acknowledgments

This work was supported by Fundação para a Ciência e a Tecnologia (FCT) and COMPETE, QREN and FEDER (PTDC/SAU-OSM/102239/2008). Authors would like to thank Dr. M. A. Vieira-Coelho (Department of Pharmacology and Therapeutics, Faculty of Medicine of Porto) for the generous gift of the prebiotics.

References

Asai, T., Hayashi, T., Kuroki, K., Okano, M., Kiriyama, T. & Kawai, T. (2011). In vitro biocompatibility of dextrin: the addition of a low concentration of dextrin in the medium promotes the cell activity of L929 mouse fibroblasts. *Cell Biol Int*, *35*, 645-8.

Balakrishnan, M. & Floch, M. H. (2012). Prebiotics, probiotics and digestive health. *Curr Opin Clin Nutr Metab Care*, *15*, 580-85.

Bradford, M. M. (1976). A rapid and sensitive method for the quantitation of microgram quantities of protein utilizing the principle of protein-dye binding. *Anal Biochem*, *72*, 248–54.

Canani, R. B., Di Costanzo, M., Leone, L., Pedata, M., Meli, R. & Calignano, A. (2011). Potential beneficial effects of butyrate in intestinal and extraintestinal diseases. *World J Gastroenterol*, *17*, 1519-28.

Cuff, M., Dyer, J., Jones, M. & Shirazi-Beechey, S. (2005). The human colonic monocarboxylate transporter isoform 1: its potential importance to colonic tissue homeostasis. *Gastroenterol*, *128*, 676–86.

Cuff, M. A., Lambert, D. W. & Shirazi-Beechey, S. P. (2002). Substrate-induced regulation of the human colonic monocarboxylate transporter, MCT1. *J Physiol*, *539*, 361–71.

Davie, J. R. (2004). Inhibition of histone deacetylase activity by butyrate. *J Nutr*, *133*, Suppl 7, 2485S-2493S.

Eiwegger, T., Stahl, B., Haidl, P., Schmitt, J., Boehm, G., Dehlink, E., Urbanek, R. & Szépfalusi, Z. (2010). Prebiotic oligosaccharides: In vitro evidence for gastrointestinal epithelial transfer and immunomodulatory properties. *Pediatr Allergy Immunol*, *21*, 1179–88.

Frank, D. N., St Amand, A. L., Feldman, R. A., Boedeker, E. C., Harpaz, N. & Pace, N. R. (2007). Molecular-phylogenetic characterization of microbial community imbalances in human inflammatory bowel diseases. *Proc Natl Acad Sci USA*, *104*, 13780-5.

Ganapathy, V., Thangaraju, M., Prasad, P. D., Martin, P. M. & Singh, N. (2013). Transporters and receptors for short-chain fatty acids as the molecular link between colonic bacteria and the host. *Curr Opin Pharmacol*, *13*, 869-74.

Gibson, G. R., Probert, H. M., Loo, J. V., Rastall, R. A., & Roberfroid, M.B. (2004). Dietary modulation of the human colonic microbiota: updating the concept of prebiotics. *Nutr Res Rev*, *17*, 259-75.

Gonçalves, P., Araújo, J. R. & Martel, F. (2011b). Characterization of butyrate uptake by nontransformed intestinal epithelial cell lines. *J Memb Biol*, *240*, 35-46.

Gonçalves, P., Gregório, I., Araújo, J. R. & Martel, F. (2012). The effect of clotrimazole on energy substrate uptake and carcinogenesis in intestinal epithelial cells. *AntiCancer Drugs*, *23*, 220–9.

Gonçalves, P., Gregório, I., Catarino, T. A. & Martel, F. (2013). The effect of oxidative stress upon the intestinal epithelial uptake of butyrate. *Eur J Pharmacol*, *699*, 88–100.

Gonçalves, P., Gregório, I. & Martel, F. (2011a). The short-chain fatty acid butyrate is a substrate of breast cancer resistance protein. *Am J Physiol Cell Physiol*, *301*, C984–C994.

Gupta, N., Martin, P. M., Prasad, P. D. & Ganapathy, V. (2006). SLC5A8 (SMCT1)-mediated transport of butyrate forms the basis for the tumor suppressive function of the transporter. *Life Sci*, *78*, 2419–25.

Hamer, H. M., Jonkers, D., Venema, K., Vanhoutvin, S., Troost, F. J. & Brummer, R.J. (2008). The role of butyrate on colonic function. *Alim Pharmacol Ther*, *27*, 104–19.

Jakobsen, C. A., Paerregaard, A., Munkholm, F. & Wewer, V. (2013). Environmental factors and risk of developing paediatric inflammatory bowel disease - a population based study 2007-2009. *J Crohns Colit*, *7*, 79-88.

Jemal, A., Siegel, R., Xu, J. & Ward, E. (2010). Cancer statistics, 2010. *CA Cancer J Clin*, *60*, 277-300.

Kirat, D., Kondo, K., Shimada, R. & Kato, S. (2009). Dietary pectin up-regulates monocaboxylate transporter1 in the rat gastrointestinal tract. *Exp Physiol*, *94*, 422–33.

Kosmus, C. E. P, Moura, E., Serrão, M. P., Real, H., Guimarães, J. T., Guedes-de-Pinho, P., Duarte, B. P., Marques, F., Martins, M. J. & Vieira-Coelho, M. A. (2011). Influence of dietary supplementation with dextrin or oligofructose on the hepatic redox balance in rats. *Mol Nutr Food Res*, *55*, 1735-9.

Lefranc-Millot, C. (2008). NUTRIOSEs 06: a useful soluble dietary fibre for added nutritional value. *Nutr Bull*, *33*, 234–9.

Loftus, E. V. Jr. (2004). Clinical epidemiology of inflammatory bowel disease: Incidence, prevalence, and environmental influences. *Gastroenterol*, *126*, 1504-17.

Miyauchi, S., Gopal, E., Fei, Y. J. & Ganapathy, V. (2004). Functional identification of SLC5A8, a tumor suppressor down-regulated in colon cancer, as a Na^+-coupled transporter for short-chain fatty acids. *J Biol Chem*, *279*, 13293-96.

Niness, K. R. (1999). Inulin and oligofructose: what are they? *J Nutr*, *129*, 1402S–1406S.

Quigley, E. M. (2012). Prebiotics and probiotics: their role in the management of gastrointestinal disorders in adults. *Nutr Clin Pract*, *27*, 195-200.

Roberfroid, M. B. (2007). Inulin-type fructans: functional food ingredients. *J Nutr*, *137*, 2493S–2502S.

Shoaf, K., Mulvey, G. L., Armstrong, G. D. & Hutkins, R. W. (2006). Prebiotic galactooligosaccharides reduce adherence of enteropathogenic Escherichia coli to tissue culture cells. *Infect Immun*, *74*, 6920-8.

Sokol, H., Seksik, P., Furet, J. P., Firmesse, O., Nion-Larmurier, I., Beaugerie, L., Cosnes, J., Corthier, G., Marteau, P. & Doré, J. (2009). Low counts of Faecalibacterium prausnitzii in colitis microbiota. *Inflamm Bowel Dis*, *15*, 1183-9.

Topping, D. L. & Clifton, P. M. (2001). Short-chain fatty acids and human colonic function: roles of resistant starch and nonstarch polysaccharides. *Physiol Rev*, *81*, 1031-64.

van den Heuvel, E. G., Wils, D., Pasman, W. J., Bakker, M., Saniez, M. H. & Kardinaal, A. F. (2004). Short-term digestive tolerance of different doses of NUTRIOSE FB, a food dextrin, in adult men. *Eur J Clin Nutr*, *58*, 1046–55.

Wang, T., Cai, G., Qiu, Y., Fei, N., Zhang, M., Pang, X., Jia, W., Cai, S. & Zhao, L. (2012). Structural segregation of gut microbiota between colorectal cancer patients and healthy volunteers. *ISME J*, *6*, 320-9.

Young, G. P., Hu, Y., Leu, R. K. & Nyskohus, L. (2005). Dietary fibre and colorectal cancer: a model for environment - gene interactions. *Mol Nutr Food Res*, *49*, 571-84.

Zenhom, M., Hyder, A., de Vrese, M., Heller, K. J., Roeder, T. & Schrezenmeir, J. (2011). Prebiotic oligosaccharides reduce proinflammatory cytokines in intestinal Caco-2 cells via activation of PPARγ and peptidoglycan recognition protein 3. *J Nutr*, *141*, 971-7.

In: Dietary Fiber
Editor: Marvin E. Clemens
ISBN: 978-1-63463-655-1
© 2015 Nova Science Publishers, Inc.

Chapter 4

EVOLUTIONARY ROLES OF DIETARY FIBER IN SUCCEEDING METABOLIC SYNDROME (MetS) AND ITS RESPONSES TO A LIFESTYLE MODIFICATION PROGRAM: A BRAZILIAN COMMUNITY-BASED STUDY

Kátia Cristina Portero McLellan [1,2,3]***,***
Fernanda Maria Manzini Ramos [1]***, José Eduardo Corrente*** [1]***,***
Lance A Sloan [2] ***and Roberto Carlos Burini*** [1]
[1]São Paulo State University/ UNESP School of Medicine, Botucatu, SP, Brasil
[2]Texas Institute for Kidney and Endocrine Disorders, Lufkin, TX, US
[3]Stephen F Austin State University, Human Sciences, Food, Nutrition and Dietetics, Nacogdoches, TX, US

ABSTRACT

Background: It is thought that our genomic heritage from late Paleolithic man, 40,000 – 100,000 years ago, influenced not only our phenotype, but also our physiological functions. Our ancestors, for approximately 84,000 generations, survived on a regimen in which plants constituted from 50 to 80% of their diet. Later during the Neolithic agricultural period, our ancestors increased fiber intake even more to amounts that would have exceeded 100g/day. Thereafter, the industrial and agro business eras (200 years ago), and the digital age (2 generations ago) have distanced the nutrition from its primate and Paleolithic ancestors. It is known that fiber, and its sources, whole grain, fruits, and vegetables are also rich in minerals, vitamins, phenolic compounds, phytoestrogens, and related antioxidants. Thus, in conjunction with the discordance between our ancient genetically determined biology and the nutritional, cultural, and activity patterns in contemporary populations that adopted the "western lifestyle", many of the so-called disease of our time have emerged. Consumption of grain products milled from all edible components of grains, have been inversely associated with mortality from a number of chronic diseases.

Objective: To find the determinants of dietary fiber intake and its role in metabolic syndrome (MetS) in a community based intervention.

Design: It was a cross-sectional study of the relationship of ingested fibers with demographic, socieconomic, anthropometric, overall health perception, and specific pathognomonic markers for obesity and MetS and each of its components. The analysis came from baseline data obtained from participants of both sexes, over 35 years of age, enrolled during the 2007-2013 period (n= 605), in the ongoing dynamic cohort, Botucatu longitudinal study "Move for health" and conducted by professionals from the Nutritional and Exercise Metabolism Centre (CeMENutri) of the Botucatu Medical School (SP, Brazil).

Results: Even in the highest quartile, dietary fiber was far below the daily recommended intake, along with its source of fruits, vegetables, and whole grains. The quartile distribution of dietary fiber intake was not influenced by any of the study variables (demographic, socieconomic, anthropometric, overall health perception, or specific pathognomonic markers for obesity and MetS); however, in association-designed studies we had found that low dietary fiber intake and its sources represent a risk factor for insulin resistance, high-blood pressure and the presence of MetS. Moreover, in longitudinal studies with lifestyle changing (LISC) interventions, we noted a faster resolution of MetS when individuals met the recommended daily dietary fiber intake than only with LISC isolated.

Conclusion: Overall individuals had a high caloric diet and a low intake of all sources of fiber. These results were irrespective to age, gender, literacy and economic reasons, probably cultural, what makes the solution more difficult. However, when these subjects were enrolled in intervention programs with LISC it was found that adding dietary fiber to the diet was an effective booster for faster resolution of MetS. Therefore, the diet adequacy of fiber seems to work by diluting the energy intake that would potentiate the higher energy expenditure of physical exercise in promoting weight (body fat) loss, along with insulin sensitivity, vasodilation, lower inflammation states, etc.

Keywords: Fiber intake, fruits and vegetables, community nutrition, metabolic syndrome, lifestyle modification

RATIONALE

In Darwin's theory of evolution it can be assumed that the process of natural selection favored those individuals who had the ability to utilize the available food supply. The Homo sapiens and his predecessors had just two primary sources of food, animal and plants. From the emergence of the human genu, Homo, about 2.4 million years ago, our ancestors, for approximately 84,000 generations, survived as hunter-gatherers, a regimen in which plants constitute from 50 to 80% of their diet. Food plants were obtained from 50 to 100 individual species of fruits and vegetables over a year's time, and dietary fiber would have exceeded 100g/day.

It is thought that our genome heritage from late Paleolithic man, 40,000 – 100,000 years ago, influenced not only our phenotype, but also our physiological functions. New genetic changes have not had the time to evolve significantly, given an estimated rate of nuclear DNA spontaneous mutation of 0.5% per million years. In the nutritional field nutrients and bioactive food components can modify epigenetic phenomena and alter the expression of genes at the transcriptional level. Folate, Vitamin B-12, Methionine, Choline, and Betaine can affect DNA methylation and histone methylation through altering 1-carbon metabolism (Choi et al., 2010, Uekawa et al., 2009). Bioactive food components directly affect enzymes. For instance, genistein and tea catechin affects DNA methyltransferases (Dunit), resveratrol, butyrate, sulforaphane and diallyl sulfide inhibit HDAC, and curcumin inhibits histone acetyl transferases (HAT) (Canani et al. 2011). In conjunction with this discordance between our ancient genetically determined biology and the nutritional, cultural, and activity patterns in contemporary western populations, many of the so-called disease of civilization have emerged and among them the modern nutrition related diseases.

Two important events have changed the course of our nutritional history: the agricultural revolution with the raising of livestock within the past 7000 – 8000 years, and more recently, the industrial revolution and its subsequent effect on nutrition during the 19th century.

The agricultural domestication era (about 350 generations) in the Neolithic period when population density reached the point that hunting for game and wild plant foods became difficult or impossible, made the utilization of cereals attractive. Actual crop cultivation followed, and in most areas, cereal became staples. Increasing dependence on cereal grains as an energy source decreased dietary consumption of fruits and vegetables by 20% or less of total energy intake.

The fiber available from rice and wheat is predominantly insoluble while that from fruits and vegetables is mainly soluble. Hence while total fiber intake probably changed little from hunter gatherers, in the Neolithic period it generally increased the insoluble/soluble dietary fiber ratio. In addition, people began to eat more vitamin-poor starches like wheat and corn. No other free-living primates routinely consume cereal grains. Evidences suggest that vegetables and fruits have more cancer-preventing potential than grains. This probably reflects the phytochemical context of fruits and vegetables. Also, fruits and vegetables could help to reduce energy intake by promoting satiety due to the high water and fiber content (Rolls et al. 2004; Tohill et al. 2004).

Seven generations further (200 years ago) the industrial era and agrobusiness have distanced even more the nutrition from its primate and Paleolithic ancestors. Roller-milling has reduced the fiber content of cereal grain-based foods so that total fiber intake has decreased to levels much below those of agriculturalists, and hunter-gatherer primates. The low intake of fiber and its sources whole grain, fruits, and vegetables continued with the digital age (2 generations ago).

It is known that whole grains are rich source of fiber, minerals (Mg, K, phosphorus, Se, Mn, Zn and Fe) vitamins (especially, B complex and E), phenolic compounds, phytoestrogens (lignans), and related antioxidants. Consumption of grain products milled from all edible components of grains has been inversely associated with mortality, incidence of diabetes, and ischemic heart disease.

The modern diet, which is inadequate when compared with the metabolic potential of our digestive system, is probably one of the causes of the increase in the number of chronic diseases and “illnesses” of the current era. There is a close correlation between nutrition and the recent exponential increase in the conditions of obesity, dyslipidemia, diabetes, hypertension, and cardiovascular disease, as seen in nations who adopted the “western lifestyle”. Evidences suggest an inverse association between dietary fiber intake and the prevalence of metabolic syndrome (MetS). Dietary interventions focusing on meeting the current recommendation of dietary fiber intake (minimum of 25g/d) through a diet rich in whole grains, fruit, and vegetables might provide many health benefits including decreasing the risk of obesity, MetS, and type 2 diabetes.

Objective

To find the determinants of dietary fiber intake and its role in MetS in a community based intervention.

Subjects and Methods

The data were obtained from the ongoing dynamic cohort (Botucatu longitudinal study – "Move for Health") and conducted by professionals from the Nutritional and Exercise Metabolism Centre (CeMENutri). The participants (over 35 years of age) come to CeMENutri spontaneously or by physician recommendations looking for preventive care or changing behavior through diet and/or physical activities. Upon registration, the subjects are submitted to baseline assessment for demography, socioeconomics, anthropometry, dietary, physical activity and fitness, postural and blood analysis. From that, they chose follow-up interventions of daily supervised exercises (strength/ jogging/ hydro) combined with dietary interventions. Clinical, anthropometric, fitness, dietary and plasma biochemical assessments were performed at baseline (M0) and every 10 weeks thereafter. All individuals were accessed for their health status (poor, regular, good, very good, excellent).

Anthropometric assessment consisted of measuring body weight and height, according to the previously described procedures (WHO 1995), followed by body mass index (BMI) estimation. Waist circumference (WC) was measured by a non-extensible and non-elastic millimeter-graded measuring tape. Measurement was made on the mid-point between the last intercostal space and the iliac crest. The reference values proposed by NCEP-ATP III (2001, 2002), were used and WC larger than 88 cm for females and 102 for males was considered to be increased. 24h dietary recall was used to assess food intake (Fisberg et al. 2005). Dietary data obtained in homemade measurements were converted into grams and milliliters to permit chemical analysis of food intake. The centesimal composition of foods was calculated using NutWin® (2002) software, version 1.5. Foods not found in the software were added from diverse composition tables and food labels (NEPA 2004, Philippi 2002). Diet quality was evaluated using the Adapted Healthy Eating Index (HEI) (Mota et al. 2008) and evaluated groups were based on portions recommended by the Adapted Food Pyramid (Philippi et al. 1999).

Systolic and diastolic arterial blood pressure was evaluated with the individual in the seated position according to the procedures described by the V Brazilian Guidelines on Arterial Hypertension (V Diretrizes Brasileiras de Hipertensao Arterial, 2005). Values of systolic blood pressure $\geq$130 mm Hg and/or diastolic blood pressure $\geq$85 mm Hg were considered abnormal.

For laboratory analyses, the individuals were submitted to blood sample collections after overnight fasting (8 a 12 hours) by standard venipuncture. Glucose, triglycerides (TG), and high-density lipoprotein cholesterol (HDL-c) concentrations were quantified in serum by the dry chemistry method. The classification of normality levels followed NCEP-ATPIII (2001, 2002).

Individuals were diagnosed as having MetS according to NCEP-ATP III (2001, 2002), with glycemia levels adapted for 100mg/dL (Grundy et al. 2006). In addition to hyperglycemia, hypertriglyceridemia (TG $\geq$ 150 mg/dL), reduced plasma levels of HDL-cholesterol (<40 for men and <50 for women), increased waist circumference and hypertension were identified as MetS components. The diagnosis of MetS is made with the presence of three or more components.

All participants were submitted to supervised exercise 5 times a week. Physical activity was accessed by the International Physical Activity Questionnaire (Craig et al. 2003), and it was classified as low, moderate and high physical activity level according to Guidelines for Data Processing and Analysis of the International Physical Activity Questionnaire (IPAQ)–Short and Long Forms.

Table 1. Socioeconomic and demographic characteristics of individuals

	n (%)
Gender	
Men	121 (20.0)
Women	482 (80.0)
Age (years)	
< 60	402 (66.6)
≥ 60	201 (33.4)
Income (minimum wages*)	
<2	107 (17.7)
2-5	339 (56.3)
6-10	130 (21.6)
11-20	22 (3.6)
>20	5 (0.8)
Education	
No education	6 (1)
Uncompleted elementary school	191 (31.7)
Completed elementary school	67 (11.1)
Uncompleted high school	15 (2.5)
Completed high school	176 (29.2)
Uncompleted college	14 (2.3)
Completed college	134 (22.2)
Health status	
Poor	43 (7.1)
Regular	194 (32.1)
Good	301 (49.8)
Very good	42 (6.9)
Excellent	25 (4.1)

* 1 minimum wage ≈ U$ 300.00.

Table 2. Characteristics of individuals according to fiber intake quartiles

	G1 (P25)	G2 (P50)	G3 (P75)	p-value
Gender (n and %)				
Men	18 (12)	25 (16.56)	28 (18.54)	0.2785
Women	132 (88)	126 (83.44)	123 (81.46)	
Age, years (n and %)				
< 60	94 (62.67)	101 (66.89)	101 (66.89)	0.6737
≥ 60	56 (37.33)	50 (33.11)	50 (33.11)	
Income, minimum wages*(n and %)				
<2	28 (18,67)	30 (19.87)	21 (13.91)	0.2304
2-5	97 (64.67)	84 (55.63)	85 (56.29)	
6-10	21 (14)	29 (19.21)	40 (26.49)	
11-20	3 (2)	6 (3.97)	4 (2.65)	
>20	1 (0.67)	2 (1.32)	1 (0.66)	
Education (number and %)				
No education	5 (3.33)	0 (0.00)	0 (0.00)	0.1494
Uncompleted elementary school	60 (40)	44 (29.14)	53 (35.10)	
Completed elementary school	16 (10.67)	21 (13.91)	16 (10.60)	
Uncompleted high school	2 (1.33)	3 (1.99)	3 (1.99)	
Completed high school	41 (27.33)	51 (33.77)	42 (27.81)	
Uncompleted college	2 (1.33)	3 (1.99)	3 (1.99)	
Completed college	24 (16)	29 (19.21)	34 (22.52)	
BMI (mean and SD)	30.28 (±5.50)	30.49 (±6.40)	31.18 (±5.81)	0.3871
WC (mean and SD)				
Men	103.74 (±3.82)	102.78(±3.31)	110.24 (±3.18)	0.2223
Women	95.39 (±1.09)	95.62 (±1.11)	96.95 (±1.13)	0.5660
Glucose (mean and SD)	101.25 (±38.03)	102.95 (±38.42)	103.41 (±30.70)	0.8438
HDL-c (mean and SD)				
Men	50.25 (±2.68)[a]	38.87 (±2.40)[b]	36.24 (±2.03)[b]	0.0005
Women	52.09 (±1.24)	50.73 (±1.27)	52.54 (±1.41)	0.5991
Triglycerides (mean and SD)	153.68 (±76,03)	173.52 (±149.9)	163.59 (±88.74)	0.2088
SBP(mean and SD)	127.84 (±19.01)	123.21 (±17.37)	127.46 (±16.98)	0.9640
DBP(mean and SD)	80 (±9.61)	79.18 (±9.89)	79.94 (±9.14)	0.5654

BMI = Body Mass Index; HDL-c = High Density Lipoprotein Cholesterol; WC = Waist Circumference; MetS = Metabolic Syndrome.

RESULTS

Cross-sectional analysis from baseline data obtained during the 2007-2013 period (n= 605), found 80% females and 66.7% under 60 years of age, 43.4% with low education (elementary or less), 74.1% living on low income (5 minimum wages or less), and 39.2% reporting regular/bad health status (self-reported) (Table 1).

The dietary fiber intake was 7.2±2.5 g/d in the lower quartile, 14.1±2.0 g/d in the mid quartile, and 25.7±8.8 g/d in the higher quartile. There were no distinction between gender or age, neither among education, income, health self-perception and physical activity status (Table 2 and Table 3).

Table 3. Health status, physical activity, body composition, clinical and biochemical characteristics of individuals according to fiber intake quartiles

	G1 (P25)	G2 (P50)	G3 (P75)	p-value
Health status				
Poor	11 (7.33)	9 (5.96)	15 (9.93)	0.8128
Regular	56 (37.33)	46 (30.46)	46 (30.46)	
Good	68 (45.33)	80 (52.98)	73 (48.34)	
Very good	9 (6.00)	11 (7,28)	10 (6.62)	
Excellent	6 (4.00)	5(3.31)	7 (4.64)	
Physical Activity				
Low	43 (29.05)	49 (32.89)	35 (23.33)	0.3730
Moderate	82 (55.41)	74 (49.66)	91 (60.67)	
High	23 (15.54)	26 (17.45)	24 (16)	
BMI				
Normal	25 (16.67)	29 (19.46)	22 (14.67)	0.3178
Overweight	55 (36.67)	48 (32.21)	42 (28)	
Obese	70 (46.67)	72 (48.32)	86 (57.33)	
WC				
Normal	46 (30.87)	57 (38.26)	38 (25.85)	0.0696
Elevated	103 (69.13)	92 (61.74)	109 (74.15)	
Glucose				
Normal	81 (71.05)	81 (72.97)	64 (64.65)	0.3945
Elevated	33 (28.95)	30 (27.03)	35 (35.35)	
HDL-c				
Normal	55 (52.38)	53 (50)	43 (46.24)	0.6867
Abnormal	50 (47.62)	53 (50)	50 (53.76)	
Triglycerides				
Normal	61 (59.80)	60 (58.25)	48 (51.61)	0.4767
Elevated	41 (40.20)	43 (41.75)	45 (48.39)	
Hypertension				
Yes	60 (53.57)	42 (40.00)	53 (51.96)	0.0964
No	52 (46.43)	63 (60.00)	49 (48.04)	
MetS				
Yes	44 (63.77)	54 (68.35)	33 (55.93)	0.3241
No	25 (36.23)	25 (31.65)	26 (44.07)	

BMI = Body Mass Index; HDL-c = High Density Lipoprotein Cholesterol; WC = Waist Circumference; MetS = Metabolic Syndrome.

Table 4. Dietary characteristics (mean value and standard deviation) of individuals according to fiber intake quartiles

	G1 (P25)	G2 (P50)	G3 (P75)	p-value
Fibers, g/day (25g-F, 38g-M)*	7.2 + _2.5[a]	14.1 + _2.0[b]	25.7 + _8.8[c]	0.0001
Energy, kcal/day	1250 + _519[a]	1543 + _552[b]	1800 + _712[b]	0.0001
Fruit, servings/day(3-5) *	0.73 + _1.2[a]	1.7 + _1.7[b]	3.1 + _2.6[c]	0.0001
Vegetables, servings/day (4-5)*	1.2 + _1.3[a]	1.6 + _2.0[b]	2.6 + _3.4[c]	0.0001
Whole grains, servings /d (5-9)*	2.6 + _1.4[a]	3.5 + _1.7[b]	4.1 + _2.4[b]	0.0001

*DRI/Brazilian Guide.

Dietary fiber intake did not seem to influence the prevalence of obesity, metabolic syndrome, and any of its components (waist circumference, blood pressure, plasma glucose, triglycerides or HDL-cholesterol) (Table 2 and 3).

The statistical differences among dietary fiber intake in the quartiles were followed by all its sources but not by the total energy intake, differentiated only by the top quartile (Table 4). Subjects in the higher quartile of fiber showed an energy intake 30.6% higher than the ones in the lower quartile.

DISCUSSION

Data from this cross-sectional community based study shows a dietary behavior pattern characterized by low fiber intake from all of its sources. Generally, people that eat more fiber tend to have a higher caloric intake; however, there were no discriminatory effects of fiber intake on either obesity or metabolic syndrome markers in the present study. Similarly, the fiber intake quartiles had no significant influences from demographic, and socioeconomic factors and health or physical activity status of the participants.

Most fruit and vegetables are low in energy density due to the high water and fiber content. Water is the food component that has the greatest impact on energy density (Grunwald et al. 2001), and when incorporated it to a meal, keeping the macronutrients and energy constant, increases satiety and decreases energy intake in a subsequent meal (Rolls et al. 1999). Fiber also reduces energy density but in a smaller proportion than water. Adding fruit and vegetables to the diet, therefore would enhance satiety, reduce energy density (Poppitt et all 1996, Rolls et al. 2000, Yao & Roberts 2001), and allow consumption of satisfying portions, resulting in reduced the caloric intake and improved weight management.

There is a substantial amount of evidence that nutrients contained in fruits and vegetables such as fiber, antioxidant vitamins, and minerals are associated with low risk of cardiovascular diseases. Our previous publication showed that an adequate intake of fruits and a traditional pattern of diet represent protective factors against metabolic syndrome (Oliveira et al. 2012, Marsola et al. 2011). Higher risk for abdominal obesity was found in individuals with low fruit intake (Castanho et al. 2013). High-plasma triglycerides were associated with lower dietary fiber intake, as well as low daily intake of whole grain, fruit or vegetables (Takahashi et al. 2010). Low dietary fiber intake was independent predictor of altered HOMA-IR. The lower consumption of fruits and higher consumption of refined grains were associated with the highest quartile of HOMA-IR (Mota et al. 2009). Diastolic pressure correlated negatively with the dietary fiber intake (Oliveira et al. 2012). In summary, our preliminary data showed that the MetS components seem to be associated with diets that are low in dietary fiber, fruits, vegetables, and whole grains.

Interestingly, the present data do not confirm these previous findings as there were no differences seen for obesity and metabolic syndrome's prevalence among the quartiles of dietary fiber intake. This finding may be attributable to the statistical approach and the data may not be comparable. Another explanation for this finding is the persistent monotonous diet, rich in calories, but poor in quality and dietary fiber from all sources, consumed by all individuals. The reason for that dietary behavior was not related to age, gender, literacy and economic status, but might be cultural, which makes the solution more difficult.

Studies have shown an association of fruit and vegetable intake on weight status, and with lifestyle and demographic factors, such as age, race, education, physical activity, smoking, intake of fat and red meet, intake of wine, multivitamins, dairy products, and fiber (Serdula et al. 1996, Trudeau et al. 1998, Liu et al. 2000). People who have a high fiber diet with large amounts of fruits and vegetables may have other lifestyle factors such as being more physically active, less likely to smoke, and consume less saturated fat, which could reduce their risk of cardiovascular disease (Serdula et al. 1996); whereas, others may use higher amounts of oil to cook their food and deep fry vegetables which will contribute to increased energy intake.

The recommended daily intake of fresh fruit and vegetables is at least 400 to 500 g/d, which means 5 servings (standard serving size) of fruits and/or vegetables a day (FAO/WHO 2003). Current international recommendations propose the intake of a minimum of 400g of fruit and vegetables (excluding potatoes and other starchy tubers) per person per day, yet most populations are not meeting this recommendation (Lock et al. 2004, FAOStat Database 2004), including the Brazilian population. The adapted Brazilian Healthy Eating Index has established a minimum and maximum recommendation intake for fruits (3 to 5 servings), vegetables (4 to 5 servings), legumes (1 serving), and whole grains (5 to 9 servings) (Mota et al. 2008). It is noted in the present study that our population consume fruits, vegetables, legumes, and whole grains far below the minimum recommended amount. Even the highest quartile of dietary fiber intake does not achieve these recommendations. Individuals in the highest quartile of fiber consumed 25.7±8.8g of dietary fiber per day, which is ineffective to reduce the risk of cardiovascular disease, diabetes, obesity, and some cancers. Our studies set a recommended dietary fiber intake goal as 25g/day, even thought studies have shown that the intake of at least 30g of fiber is necessary to obtain health benefits (Bernaud et al. 2013).

Our long term intervention studies with lifestyle changing (LISC) show a faster resolution of MetS when a high fiber diet is associated with endurance and/or resistance aerobic exercises. When the intervention was focusing on meeting the recommended dietary fiber intake (25g/d) with a physical exercise program, we noted a 24% reduction of MetS after 10 weeks (Mecca et al. 2012). Moreover, decreasing dietary fiber intake after the 6 months intervention with LISC was one of the predicted risk factors for the MetS appearance (Burini 2011). Therefore, the strategy to limit energy consumption by adding dietary fiber to the diet in association with a exercise-training protocol has shown to be an alternative for a MetS regression.

CONCLUSION

Overall individuals had a high caloric and low fiber diet from all dietary sources. These results were not associated with age, gender, literacy, and economic status, and maybe probably cultural, which makes the solution more difficult. However, when these subjects were enrolled in longitudinal studies, we found that the recommended dietary fiber intake in association with LISC accelerated the resolution of MetS. Therefore, adequate dietary fiber intake decreases the caloric density of the diet, which, in addition to higher energy expenditure from physical exercise promote fat and weight loss.

ACKNOWLEDGMENTS

Special thanks to the Brazilian Research Funding FAPESP (partial financial support) and CNPq (RCB fellowship).

REFERENCES

Bernaud FSR, Rodrigues TC. Fibra Alimentar – Ingestão adequada e efeitos sobre a saúde do metabolismo. *Arq Bras Endocrinol Metabol* 2013; 57(6): 397-405.

Burini FHP. *Resposta dos componentes da síndrome metabólica a programa de mudança do estilo de vida em adultos*. 2011. Tese (Doutorado em Interunidades em Nutrição Humana Aplicada) - Universidade de São Paulo.

Canani RB, Costanzo MD, Leone L, Bedogni G, Brambilla P, Cianfarani S, et al. Epigenetic mechanisms elicited by nutrition in early life. *Nutr Res Rev*. 2011;24(2):198-205.

Castanho GKF, Marsola FC, Mclellan KCP, Nicola M, Burini RC. Consumo de frutas, verduras e legumes associado à Síndrome Metabólica e seus componentes em amostra populacional adulta. *Ciência e Saúde Coletiva* 2013;18:385-392.

Choi AW, Friso S. *Epigenetics: A New Bridge between Nutrition and Health.* Adv Nutr 2010; 1: 8-16.

Diet, nutrition and the prevention of chronic diseases. Report of a joint FAO/WHO Expert Consultation, World Health Organization, 2003 (WHO Techinical Report Series, No. 916).

Executive Summary of The Third Report of The National Cholesterol Education Program (NCEP) Expert Panel on Detection, Evaluation, And Treatment of High Blood Cholesterol In Adults (Adult Treatment Panel III). *JAMA* 2001, 285:2486-2497.

FAOStat Database, *Food and Agriculture Organization,* Rome, 2004.

Fisberg RM, Slater B, Marchioni DML, Martini LA: *Inquéritos Alimentares - Métodos e Bases Científicos.* Barueri: Manole 2005.

Grundy SM: Metabolic syndrome: connecting and reconciling cardiovascular and diabetes worlds. *J Am Coll Cardiol* 2006, 47:1093-1100.

Grunwald GK, Seagle HM, Peters JC, Hill JO. Quantifying and separating the effects of macronutrient composition and non-macronutrientes on energy density. *Br J Nutr* 2001, 86:265-276.

Institute of Medicine. *Dietary Reference Intakes: Energy, Carbohydrate, Fiber, Fat, Fatty Acids, Cholesterol, Protein, and Amino Acids.* Washington, D.C., National Academics Press; 2005.

Liu S, Manson AE, Lee IM, Cole SH, Hennekens CH, Willett WC et al. Fruit and vegetable intake and risk of cardiovascular disease: the Woman's Healthy Study. *Am J Clin Nutr* 2000, 72:922-928.

Lock K, Pomerleau J, Causer L, McKee M. Low fruit and vegetable consumption. In: Ezzati M, Lopez AD, Rodgers A, Murray CJL. *Comparative quantification of health risks: global and regional burden of disease due to selected major risk factors.* Geneva, World Health Organization, 2004.

Marsola FC, Rinaldi AEM, Siqueira M, Mclellan KCP, Corrente JE, Burini RC. Association of dietary patterns with metabolic syndrome components in low-income, free-living Brazilian adults. *Int J Nutr Metabol* 2011; 3:31-38.

Mecca M, Fernando M, Burini FHP, Dalanesi, RC, Mclellan KCP, Burini RC. Ten-week lifestyle changing program reduces several indicatiors for metabolic syndrome in overweight adults. *Diabetology & Metabolic Syndrome 2012*; 4:1.

Mello VD, Laaksonen DE. Fibras na dieta: tendências atuais e benefícios à saúde na síndrome metabólica e no diabetes melito tipo 2. *Arq Bras Endocrinol Metab* 2009; 53(5):509-518.

Mota JF, Rinaldi AEM, Pereira AF, Maestá N, Scarpin MM, Burini RC: Adaptation of the healthy eating index to the food guide of the Brazilian population. *Rev Nutri* 2008, 21:545-552.

Mota JF, Medina WL, Moreto F, Burini RC. Influência da adiposidade sobre o risco inflamatório em pacientes com glicemia de jejum alterada. *Rev Nutr* 2009, 22;351-357.

NEPA/UNICAMP: *Tabela brasileira de composição de alimentos.* Taco. Versão 1. Campinas; 2004.

Oliveira EP, Camargo KF, Castanho GKF, Nicola M, Mclellan KCP, Burini RC. A variedade da dieta é fator protetor para a pressão arterial sistólica elevada. *Arquivos Brasileiros de Cardiologia (Impresso)* 2012;1:1 - 6.

Oliveira EP, Mclellan KCP, Silveira LVA, Burini RC. Dietary factors associated with metabolic syndrome in Brazilian adults. *Nutrition Journal* 2012;11:13.

Philippi ST, Latterza AR, Cruz ATR, Ribeiro LC: Adapted food pyramid: a guide for a right food choice. *Rev Nutri* 1999, 12:65-80.

Philippi ST: *Tabela de Composição de Alimentos: Suporte para decisão nutricional.* 2ª ed. São Paulo; 2002.

Rolls BJ, Bell EA, Thorwart ML. Water incorporated into a food but not served with a food decreases energy intake in lean women. *Am J Clin Nutr* 1999, 70:448-455.

Rolls BJ, Ello-Martin JA, Tohill BC. What can intervention studies tell us about the relationship between fruit and vegetable consumption and weight management? *Nutr Rev.* 2004;62:1-17

Serdula MK, Byers T, Mokdad AH, Simoes E, Mendlein JM, Coates RJ. The association between fruit and vegetable intake and chronic disease risk factors. *Epidemiology* 1996; 7:161-165.

Takahashi MM, Oliveira EP, Moreto F, Mclellan KCP, Burini RC. Association of dyslipidemia with intakes of fruit and vegetables and the body fat content of adults clinically selected for lifestyle modification program. *Archivos Latinoamericanos de Nutrición* 2010;60:148-154.

Third Report of the National Cholesterol Education Program (NCEP) Expert Panel on Detection, Evaluation, and Treatment of High Blood Cholesterol in Adults (Adult Treatment Panel III) final report. *Circulation* 2002, 106:3143-3421.

Tohill BC, Seymour J, Serdula M, Kettel-Khan L, Rolls BJ. What epidemiologic studies tell us about the relationship between fruit and vegetable consumption and body weight. *Nutr Rev.* 2004;62(10):365-374.

Trudeau E, Kristal AR, Li S, Patterson RE. Demographic and psychosocial predictors of fruit and vegetable intakes differ: implications for dietary intervention. *J Am Diet Assoc* 1998, 98: 1412-1417.

Uekawa A, Katsushima K, Ogata A, Kawata T, Maeda N, Kobayashi K, Maekawa A, Tadokoro T, Yamamoto Y. Change of epigenetic control of cystathionine beta-synthase gene expression through dietary vitamin B12 is not recovered by methionine supplementation. *J Nutrigenet Nutrigenomics.* 2009;2:29–36.

V Diretrizes Brasileiras de Hipertensão Arterial. *Revista da Sociedade Brasileira de Cardiologia* 2005, 84.

In: Dietary Fiber
Editor: Marvin E. Clemens

ISBN: 978-1-63463-655-1
© 2015 Nova Science Publishers, Inc.

Chapter 5

ROLE OF FIBER IN DAIRY COW NUTRITION AND HEALTH

Nazir Ahmad Khan[1,2], Katerina Theodoridou[1] and Peiqiang Yu[1,3,*]
[1]Department of Animal and Poultry Science, College of Agriculture and Bioresources, University of Saskatchewan, Saskatoon, Canada
[2]Department of Animal Nutrition, The University of Agriculture, Peshawar, Pakistan
[3]Department of Animal Science, Tianjin Agricultural University, Tianjin, China

ABSTRACT

The fiber fraction of plant cell walls is one of the major sources of nutrients and energy. Mammals do not produce enzymes that can hydrolyze β1-4 linked polysaccharides (cellulose and hemicellulose) of plant cell walls, and as such fiber cannot be directly used to feed the growing global human population. By symbiosis with rumen microbes, ruminants are capable of converting this non-digestible food resource into high-quality animal products. For dairy cows, fiber is an important feed component, not only as an energy and nutrient source, but also as a regulatory factor for the maintenance of rumen health and feed intake. Compared to other nutrients, fiber, particularly forage-fiber, has much longer ruminal retention time because of slower degradation and greater buoyancy in the rumen. As such feeding fiber with large particle size can increases digesta mass in the rumen that in turn stimulate rumination, increases rumen buffering capacity and reduces the risk of ruminal acidosis and abomasal displacement. On the other hand rumen-fill can also limit feed intake, and the filling effect of fiber in more pronounced in high producing dairy cows. Any reduction in dry matter intake reduces milk and milk protein yield of dairy cows. Therefore, high producing dairy cows can be benifited from feeding fiber sources with rapid rumen-passage rate.

Legumes and corn silage fiber digests and passes from the rumen quickly compared to perennial grasses and can be an excellent source of forage fiber for high producing cows. Fiber-turnover through the rumen is influenced by many factors, these includes intrinsic plant characteristics such as fiber content, particle size, fragility (rate of particle size reduction) and digestibility (rate of fermentation), and extrinsic factors within the

* Corresponding author: Dr. Peiqiang Yu, Professor and Ministry of Agriculture Strategic Research Chair, University of Saskatchewan, Canada. Tel.: (306) 966 4132, e-mail: peiqiang.yu@usask.ca.

rumen environment, such as rumination, absorption of fermentation end products, rumen pH and growth of the microbial population. The fiber fraction generally becomes more lignified, as forage matures, and the degree of fiber lignifications is directly related to the filling effects of the fiber within a forage type. Fiber that is less lignified are more digestible and clears from the rumen faster, allowing more space for the next meal. Selecting forages with high fiber digestibility can increase their feeding value. Alternatively, lignin degrading enzymes can also improve fiber digestibility, however the effect is not consistent. Some fungi specifically degrade lignin in cell walls, and can improve fiber digestibility in low quality fibrous materials such as crop residues. Improving the intake and digestion of fiber in dairy cows will result in a more efficient conversion of this non-digestible food resource into high-quality animal products. The total digestion of fiber is the major determinant of its energy value, however, rate of digestion and physical properties play an important role in maintaining rumen health.

1. Introduction

A large part of the solar energy reaching to our planet is stored in the fiber fraction of plant cell walls. Fiber cannot be digested by endogenous mammalian enzymes, and as such a major proportion of the solar energy cannot be directly used to feed the growing global human population. By symbiosis with rumen microbes, ruminants are capable of utilizing the energy and nutrients stored in the fiber fraction of plant cell walls. Fiber has an important role in dairy cattle nutrition and health, because it is required to support an appropriate rumen function and physiology. In the wild, but also in many intensive production systems, forages are the major source of fiber in dairy cows ration. For dairy cows, forage-fiber is an important feed component, not only as a major energy source, but also as a regulator factor for feed intake, rumen pH and milk fat content. On the other hand, fiber is the least digestible (40 to 70%) component of dairy ration, whereas the digestibility of non-fiber feed component is very high (> 90%) and less variable (Mertens, 2009).

Therefore, fiber content, fiber degradability in the rumen as well as particle size and fragility are the major determinant of feed digestibility, dry matter intake (DMI) and feed efficiency in dairy cows. This background shows that understanding the optimum feeding of fiber in dairy rations is important for an efficient conversion of these non-digestible food resources into high-quality animal products.

On the one hand, feeding high proportion of forages in dairy ration is important to extract maximum energy and nutrients from fiber, reduce feed cost and ensure long-term sustainability of dairy production. On the other hand, fiber generally has a large indigestible fraction with a slower rate of particle size reduction, and the potentially degradable fraction degrades at a slower rate in the rumen. Therefore, high proportion of forages (fiber) in dairy ration can reduce energy density, DMI and milk yield of high producing dairy cows (Yang and Beauchemin, 2006). Nevertheless, providing high-producing dairy cows with adequate amount of coarse fiber from forages is critical for maintaining proper rumen functions, fiber digestion, rumen pH and milk fat content, and avoiding metabolic disorders. When too little fiber is incorporated in dairy ration, the bulkiness, chewing time and digesta mass is reduced; as a consequence less salivary buffer is produced leading to lower rumen pH and acetated production that results in reduced milk fat synthesis. The lower rumen pH also reduces fiber digestion.

This background provides an impetus to include an optimum content of dietary fiber in dairy ration. The objective of this chapter is to review (1) recent advance in fiber characterization and analysis; (2) fiber subfractions and their characteristics; (3) importance of effective fiber in dairy nutrition; (4) factors affecting fiber requirement of dairy cow and the consequences of lower and higher fiber content in dairy ration (5) factors affecting fiber degradability; and (6) to provide guidelines for optimum fiber content in dairy ration in terms of DMI, rumen health, and milk yield and composition.

2. CARBOHYDRATES IN FORAGES

From nutritional point of view, carbohydrates in forages are broadly classified into structural and non-structural carbohydrates (Figure 1). The structural carbohydrates are comprised of elements that are present in the cell walls of plants and non-structural carbohydrates are found inside the cells (Ishler and Varga, 2001).

The structural carbohydrates are incompletely digestible, whereas the nonstructural carbohydrates are usually more (completely) digestible. Plant cell walls are comprised of cellulose, hemicellulose, lignin, pectic and β-glucans. The non-structural carbohydrates contain starches, sugars, fructans, and organic acids for ensiled feeds. Pectins are considered non-structural carbohydrate because it is not covalently linked to the lignified portions of plant cell walls and are almost completely digested (90 to100 percent) in the rumen.

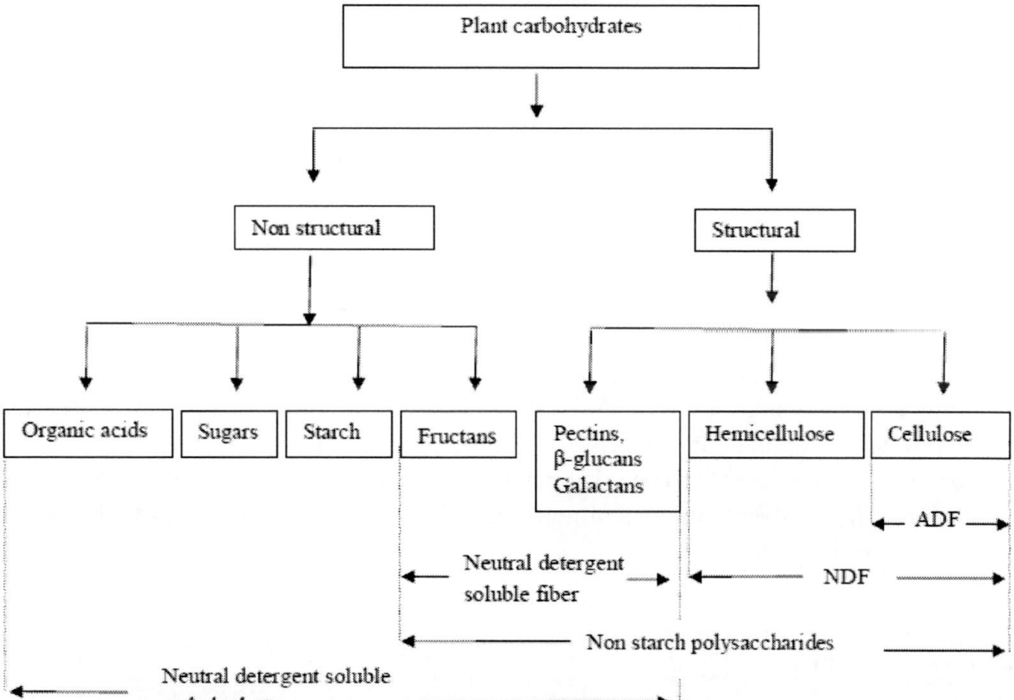

The ADF = acid detergent fiber; and the NDF = neutral detergent fiber.

Figure 1. Classification of plant carbohydrates.

Pectin contents on a DM basis are high in citrus and beet pulps, soybean hulls, and dicotyledonous legume forages, but are low in grasses (Allen, 1995).

Similarly, other completely digestible fibers such as β-glucan gums which are present in cell walls of grasses, and galactans which are present in the cell walls of leguminous plants are not included in structural carbohydrates (Aman and Hesselman, 1985). To summarize, in ruminant nutrition the structural carbohydrates include cellulose, hemicelluloses and lignin, and the non-structural carbohydrates include starches, sugars, fructans, pectins, β-glucan gums, galactans, and organic acids for ensiled feeds.

3. What Is Fiber?

In nutrition fiber refers to plant-derived food or feed component that is not digestible by mammalian enzymes (Moore and Hatfield, 1994). Mammals do not produce enzymes that can hydrolyze β1-4 linked polysaccharides (cellulose and hemicellulose) of plant cell walls, and depend on microorganisms in the gastrointestinal tract to ferment these polysaccharides to absorbable nutrients. For ruminants, both chemical and physical characteristics of fiber are important due to their influence on the mechanical processes of digestion (chewing, degradation and passage), rumen pH and animal health.

Therefore, Mertens (1997) preferred a more restrictive definition of fiber as the "indigestible and slowly digesting fractions of feed that occupies space in the gastrointestinal tract". In ruminant nutrition fiber usually refers to the insoluble components of plant cell walls, namely, cellulose, hemicellulose and lignin. Some fibers such as pectin, fructans and β-glucans are soluble in the chemicals (e.g., mild acid, detergent solutions) used for fiber extraction and thus referred as "soluble fiber".

The soluble fiber readily fermented in the rumen and may even be readily fermented in the large intestine of monogastric animals. Soluble fiber has limited role in stimulation of chewing, and maintenance of DMI, rumen pH and animal health.

3.1. Fiber Analysis

The common goal of fiber analysis is to determine its concentration in the feed. The commonly used fiber analyses in forage quality and ruminant nutrition are crude fiber, neutral detergent fiber (NDF), acid detergent fiber (ADF) and acid detergent lignin (ADL). All these methods use the traditional gravimetric principles after chemical extraction of the non-fiber components. The uses, limitations and nutrition meaning of these methods of fiber analysis are summarized in Table 1.

3.2. Crude Fiber

The proximate or Weende system of analysis (Henneberg and Stohmann, 1859) is the oldest method for the measurement of crude fiber in animal feeds. In this method, feed sample is sequentially refluxed in dilute base followed by dilute acid.

Table 1. Uses, limitations and nutrition meaning of some of the major methods of fiber

Method of analysis	Cell wall fraction	Limitations of method	Nutritional meaning
Neutral detergent fiber (NDF)	Cellulose, hemicellulose and lignin	Soluble fibers are almost completely removed Protein and starch removal can be a problem	Associated with rumen fill Correlates negatively with dry matter intake Correlates positively with rumination Correlates negatively with energy content
Acid detergent fiber (ADF)	Cellulose and lignin	A significant fraction of lignin is solubalized	Associated with net energy lactation Correlates negatively with digestibility
Acid detergent lignin	Lignin	Lignin solubalized at ADF step, especially in grasses	Correlates negatively with digestibility of NDF Unavailable NDF = 2.4 × lignin
Crude fiber	Cellulose	Noncellulosic polysaccharides such as hemicelluose and lignin are not measured	Correlates negatively with energy content of feed

The residues left after filtration is the crude fiber fraction, which was originally thought to represent the indigestible portion of feed. Later on, it was shown that it is composed primarily of cellulose and variable proportions of noncellulosic polysaccharides and lignin. The crude fiber method recovers only a fraction of cell walls and markedly underestimates the total plant fiber content. The crude fiber is an official method of AOAC, and continues to be used today because a large database has been accumulated for a wide variety of feeds.

3.3. Neutral Detergent Fiber

In ruminant nutrition, the NDF method developed by Van Soest (Van Soest, 1963; Van Soest et al., 1991) has largely replaced crude fiber. Neutral detergent fiber, like crude fiber, uses chemical extraction with a neutral detergent solution under reflux. Water and detergent soluble compounds are removed and the residue left after filtration is called NDF. The soluble compounds includes β- glucans, galactans and fructans. The insoluble fraction represents the fiber (NDF) fraction, and comprised of cellulose, hemicelluloses and lignin. However, variable amounts of ash and protein also remains with the residues. After extraction the NDF is measured gravimetrically. The NDF is considered to be the entire fiber fractionof the feed, but it is known to underestimate cell walls content because most of the soluble fibers in the cell walls are solubilized and filtered-out from the NDF residues (Van Soest, 1994). As a result, NDF gives a poor estimation of cell walls content in pectin-rich legumes. Heat-damaged proteins in processed feeds, and lignin and tannins bounded protein in mature forages are also retained in NDF, which overestimate the NDF content. Ash contamination also overestimates the NDF value. Soil contamination often is the major contributor to the ash residues.

It is recommended that NDF should be expressed on an ash, protein and starch free basis. Currently, sodium sulfite and heat-stable amylase is used to remove starch and protein contamination from NDF. This is the reference method of both National Forage Testing Association and NRC (2001). Using sodium sulfite in the NDF procedure is discouraged if the residues are to be assayed for neutral detergent insoluble protein.

Sulfite addition is also discouraged if the NDF residue has to be sequentially analyzed for lignin or in vitro digestibility. Sulfite attack lignin and does not quantitatively remove all the protein. Feeds with higher contents (> 10%) of fat such as oil seeds can give inflated values of NDF, because fat is not completely extracted from the feed.

In such situation extraction of fat, such as with a 2 h incubation in acetone, prior to NDF analysis is recommended. If fiber is defined as the incompletely digestible fraction of feeds, then the shortcomings of NDF method will be of less concern. Although widely used for fiber analysis, the NDF procedure is not an official AOAC method.

3.4. Acid Detergent Fiber

Acid detergent fiber represents the least digestible fraction of plant cell walls. The ADF procedure is an AOAC approved method, and uses acid detergent solution under reflux, for extraction of acid detergent soluble compounds. Acid detergent fiber is the residues remaining after filtration, and includes lignin and cellulose fraction of cell walls.

The ADF residues may contain ash, variable amounts of xylans and insoluble forms of nitrogen. The ADF insoluble protein is non-degradable in the rumen and indigestible in the post-ruminal tract. The ADF insoluble protein fraction is used to determine the unavailable fraction of protein in heated and high tannins containing feeds.

It is recommended to express ADF on an ash-free basis. The ADF is often used to estimate feed digestibility, total digestible nutrients and net energy for lactation.

3.5. Lignin Analysis

Lignin is a non-carbohydrate, high molecular weight compound that constitutes a diverse class of phenolic compounds. Many methods of lignin analysis have been developed because of lignin's negative association with digestibility. Acid detergent lignin is the most common method used for lignin analysis in ruminant nutrition.

According to this method feed samples are first analyzed for ADF. The ADF residues are then digested in 72% sulphuric acid for 2 h, which removes the hemicellulose from the residues. Acid detergent lignin is then determined gravimetrically.

Some lignin at the ADF step is solubalized and this is the reason for the underestimation of feed lignin content with this method (Lowry et al. 1994).

3.6. Estimation of Cellulose and Hemicellulose

In ruminant nutrition, the cellulose content of forages is commonly estimated as ADF minus ADL. Cellulose concentrations are overestimated by ADF minus ADL to the extent that xylans are present in ADF and underestimated by heat-damaged protein contamination of ADL. Whereas, the hemicellulose content of forages is commonly estimated as NDF minus ADF. The hemicellulose is overestimated by protein residues in NDF. On the other hand, xylans residues in ADF underestimate the hemicellulose.

3.7. Recent Advances in Fiber Analysis

Recently, the NDF and ADF methods have been adopted for the use semi-automated equipments, Ankom 200 Fiber Analyzer (Ankom Technology Corp., Fairport, NY; and Fibertec I, Perstorp Analytical, Silver Spring, MD), which reduces the analysis duration, and increases samples handling capacity.

Similarly, Near-infrared spectroscopy (NIRS) can be used to rapidly estimate the fiber content and composition of feed samples. The NIR is a non-destructive and non-invasive method that can directly analyze the fiber content of dried and ground forages. Near-infrared spectroscopy technology depends on the correlation of near-infrared reflectance spectra of samples with actual analytical measurements of the fiber content and composition by wet chemical analysis.

Once a reliable library is established, then NIR can rapidly analyze large number of feed samples, because it does not require the time consuming extraction process. Although many chemical entities have been successfully analyzed using NIRS, this method has limited application in fiber analysis due to the quality of the reference analytical methods and similarity of the sample to the calibrated samples.

Other molecular spectroscopic methods have been applied in feed-related biomaterial analysis which included Fourier Transform Infra-red; Diffuse Reflectance Infra-red Fourier Transform, (Jonker et al., 2012), Attenuated Total Reflectance - Fourier Transform infra-red (Yu et al., 2014; Chen et al., 2014), Raman (Yu and Zhang, 2014) and Advanced synchrotron based infrared microspectroscopy (Yu, 2004).

These molecular spectroscopic techniques have made contributions to quantify the content and composition of biopolymers such as cellulose, hemicellulose and lignin but they are still in developing stage.

4. Neutral Detergent Fiber

4.1. Importance of Neutral Detergent Fiber Content of the Diet

Among the current methods of fiber analysis, only NDF measures the total (> 90%) fiber content of feed, and quantitatively determine differences between forage families (grasses *vs.* legumes), within forage type (young *vs.* mature grasses; warm *vs.* cool season grasses), and between forages and concentrates (Mertens, 1997; Mertens, 2009).

Moreover, the NDF is better related to rumen fill and DMI than any other measurements of fiber (Van Soest et al., 1991). Thus, fiber requirements of dairy cow are better measured in terms of NDF rather than ADF or crude fiber.

4.2. Optimal NDF Level in the Diet

Formulating rations with an optimum NDF content is very challenging, because many variables such as fiber fragility (rate of particle size reduction), degradability (rate of fermentation), physical characteristics (particle size, density etc.) as well as animal's energy requirement affect NDF requirement of dairy cows (Mertens, 1997; De Brabander et al., 1999; Zebeli et al., 2006).

In addition, it is very difficult to extrapolate research data and determine a true relationship between NDF content and DMI and milk production of dairy cow to make recommendation for optimum NDF level, mainly due to the fact that research studies varies in many factors, i.e., fiber sources (forage *vs.* non-forage), forage type, stage of lactation and manner of data expression. Moreover, NDF does not account for a large portion of the variability associated with ruminal availability of fiber (NDF content *vs.* digestibility). Variation in digesta kinetics related to stage of lactation may also impact NDF digestion.

Finally, NDF is not a uniform chemical entity, but consists of cellulose, hemicellulose and lignin (indigestible fraction of NDF), which varies greatly between (e.g., grass *vs.* legumes) and within (e.g., young *vs.* mature) forages. It has been shown that the content of lignin as well as its bonding with hemicelluloses greatly affects fiber (cellulose, hemicellulose) degradability and effectiveness.

Due to lack of accurate data, the current recommendations for forage and total NDF contents of dairy rations (Table 2; NRC, 2001) are only the minimum amounts required for maintaining proper rumen function, milk fat content and animal health. The NRC (2001) recommends a minimum of 25% NDF in dairy ration, in which 19% (75% of total NDF) must be supplied by forages. As the non-forage NDF is less effective in maintaining rumen function compared to forage-NDF, the minimum amount of total NDF increases from 25% to 33% (diet DM), as the proportion of forage-NDF decreases from 19% to 15% (diet DM; Table 2). Formulating rations for NDF successfully means avoiding both deficiency and excess of NDF in dairy ration. This means NDF levels needs to be adjusted based on the characteristics of NDF sources and animal production stage, and not using one constant value for all herds.

Table 2. Recommended minimum concentrations (% of dry matter(DM) of neutral detergent fiber (NDF) from forages and total diet NDF and recommended maximum concentrations (% of DM) of non-fiber carbohydrates (NFC) for diets containing ground corn as primary starch source fed as total mixed ration of adequate particle size (NRC, 2001)

Minimum NDF from Forage	Minimum NDF in Diet	Maximum NFC in Diet[1]
19	25	44
18	27	42
17	29	40
16	31	38
15[2]	33	36

[1]NFC = 100 – ((%NDF - NDIP) + %CP + %Fat + %ash), where NDIP is neutral detergent insoluble protein

[2]Not recommended because of depression of milk fat test.

4.3. Consequences of NDF Deficiency

Rumen and dairy cow health is negatively affected by low NDF and high non-fiber carbohydrate rations. When the (effective)-NDF content is deficient in dairy ration, chewing activity and salivary buffer secretion decreases, which leads to a lower rumen pH, altered fermentation and a lower acetate to propionate ratio that results in a modified animal metabolism and lower milk fat synthesis. It can be argued that NDF deficiency in the ration may not be the primary cause of the preceding scenario. Under many dietary regimes, grains are used to replace NDF in the low NDF rations, and these rapidly fermenting carbohydrates may contribute to animal responses to low fiber rations (Mertens, 1997). Low NDF and high non-fiber carbohydrate rations results in high production of volatile fatty acids, which decreases rumen pH. At the same time the buffering capacity of the rumen is reduced by lowers buffer secretion, and lower digesta mass (less dilution) and rumen motility (less absorption). The volatile fatty acids absorption is also reduced because of lower rumen mixing and acids contact with ruminal walls. Low ruminal pH also damage papillae and causes the adhesion of adjacent papillae, which reduces the absorptive surface area, resulting in a decrease rate of volatile fatty acids removal. A general term used to describe these NDF deficiency related problems is rumen acidosis. Several indirect indicators can be used to asses if rumen acidosis is taking place. Indicators that respond quickly to NDF deficiency include a decrease in chewing time, rumen pH and milk fat content. Long-term effects include laminitis and an increased incidence of ketosis and abomasal displacement. Normally, more than one indicator should be used to make a more accurate assessment of rumen acidosis.

4.3.1. Milk Fat Percentage

There is a strong positive relationship between rumen pH and milk fat content. An abrupt drop in milk fat content may indicate low rumen pH. However, the milk fat content of early lactating high producing dairy cows is less sensitive to changes in rumen pH because they are often in negative energy balance and mobilizes their body fat. Moreover, feeding high amount of fat, particularly polyunsaturated fat, to dairy cows can reduce milk fat content.

4.3.2. Chewing Activity

During rumen acidosis the frequency of rumination decreases and the observation of normal chewing activity are often used as an indicator for rumen acidiosis. A poor relationship between chewing time and rumen pH, and variation observed in the chewing activities among healthy cows, restrict the usefulness of this indicator. However, a noticeable reduction in rumination of a number of cows for one to two hours after consuming meal can be used jointly with other indicators for assessment of rumen acidosis.

4.3.3. Changes in Dry Matter Intake

Low and irregular DMI may also indicate rumen acidosis. The knowledge of feed intakes history is necessary in order to use this indicator effectively. Feed intake is herd specific and it is affected by many factors. Therefore, routine and continuous monitoring is important to distinguish between explainable drops in feed intake and that caused by rumen acidosis.

4.3.4. Fecal Consistency

During rumen acidosis the fluidity of manure may increase. This occurs when a low NDF, high non-fiber carbohydrate diet is consumed by dairy cow, which increases lactic acid flow to the post-ruminal tract, and also in case when some starch escape ruminal fermentation and small intestinal digestion, and get fermented to volatile fatty acids in the large intestine. Both of these conditions can increase the osmolarity in large intestine causing an influx of water from the blood.

A severe change in feacal consistency in combination with other issues may be used as an indicator for ruminal acidosis.

4.3.5. Laminitis

Laminitis is an aseptic inflammation of the dermal layers inside the foot, above the hoof and around the coronary band. Cow suffering with laminitis generally moving stiffly, and standing on toes on the edge of their stall because of severe pain.

Rumen acidosis has been shown to be a major cause of laminitis.

As the rumen pH decreases below 5, acid accumulation increases in the rumen, which results in a stasis of fermentation. As a consequence endotoxins are produced, and this triggers histamine release. Histamine causes vasoconstriction, dilation, laminar destruction, hoof deterioration and the laminitis process develops.

However, histamine is also naturally released when an animal is stressed such as due to abrupt change in environment or due to the occurrence of infectious disease.

The main problem with using laminitis as an indicator is that the hemorrhage develop 2 to 3 months after the occurrence of rumen acidosis, as such it may have little relevance to the current feeding program.

4.4. What Determines the Upper Limit of NDF in Dairy Ration?

The upper limit of NDF in the ration is a function of the cow's energy requirement, the minimum amount of non-fiber carbohydrates necessary to support microbial growth and normal rumen function, and the potential negative effect of NDF on feed intake.

The NDF content of the diet usually did not constrain DMI when diets contained adequate amount of net energy for lactation. The DMI of dairy cows is reduced by rumen fill, only when they are in negative or slightly positive energy balance. During early lactation the demand for energy is high, particularly in high producing dairy cows.

Therefore excess of NDF can severely reduce DMI during early lactation as compared to mid and late lactation. The maximum NDF or minimum non-fiber carbohydrates a cow can tolerate also depends on the rates of particle size reduction of the indigestible fraction and the rate of fermentation of the potentially degradable NDF.

Feeding overly mature forages, especially grasses with excessively long particles can results in longer retention and rumen fill. Feeding of inadequate non-fiber carbohydrates can depress microbial growth, and decreases fiber digestion.

These scenarios demonstrate the importance of evaluating both the chemical and physical properties of the ration.

5. PHYSICALLY EFFECTIVE FIBER

It has been widely demonstrated that not only the amount, but also the physical form of dietary fiber is important for maintenance of proper rumen function, animal health and milk fat content in dairy cows. Neutral detergent fiber measures the chemical characteristics, but not the physical characteristics of fiber such as particle size and density. Thus, the concept of physically effective NDF (peNDF) was created to combine the chemical characteristics and particle size of forages, and to quantify its value to rumen function (Mertens, 1997). Physically effective NDF indicate that portion of dairy ration (fiber) that stimulates chewing activity and salivary buffer production, and establishes a biphasic stratification of ruminal contents i.e., a floating mat of large particles on a pool of liquid and small particles (Zebeli et al., 2005). Saliva production is important to buffer the acids produced during rumen fermentation. Rumen mat traps small feed particles that would otherwise escape rumen fermentation, and as such increases diet digestibility. Moreover, peNDF increases digesta volume which dilute fermentation acids and increases their absorption because of increased ruminal contraction. The large fiber particles also stay for longer time in the rumen, and supply consistent energy to rumen microbes and dairy cow throughout the day.

5.1. Measurement of Physically Effective Fiber

The Penn State Particle Separator (PSPS) device is commonly used to measure the peNDF content of dairy ration. The first version of PSPS separates feed particles according to their size into >19 mm, between 19 and 8 mm, and < 8 mm (Figure 2; Lammers et al., 1996). The peNDF is a measure of the proportion of DM retained by the 19 and 8 mm PSPS screens multiplied by dietary NDF content. Mertens (1997) postulated that in terms of animal performance, the peNDF is better expressed as the proportion of DM retained by the 1.18 mm screen multiplied by dietary NDF. The new version of PSPS include an additional sieve of 1.18 mm (Kononoff et al., 2003), permitting the estimation of peNDF >1.18 as proposed by Mertens (1997). An alternative approach is to avoid an index system and to evaluate peNDF by considering the NDF content and particle size of the dairy ration separately.

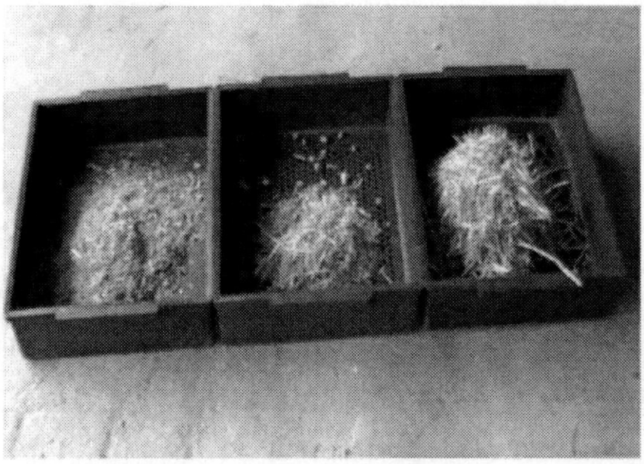

Figure 2. Penn State Particle Separator device.

5.2. Effect of Forage Particle Size on Chewing Activity

Literature data on the effect of particle size on chewing time is summarized in Table 3. The data shows that particle size reduction of forages by chopping and grinding decreases chewing activity per kilogram of DM and NDF. The magnitude of the decrease in chewing time was related to the initial particle size, the reduction in particle size and forage NDF content. The largest reduction of 79% in particle size occurred when ryegrass was finely chopped. A key question for dairy nutritionist is: what is the critical particle size for passage from the rumen, and which fraction of particles remains in the rumen to stimulate chewing, saliva production, and rumen buffering (Einarson et al., 2004). The particles greater than 1.18 mm are believed to be highly resistant to passage out of the rumen, it is speculated this fraction stimulates chewing activity. Mertens (1997) consequently adopted the 1.18 mm sieving approach to fractionate the larger feed particles requiring chewing to pass from the rumen and this 1.18 mm fraction has become the standard laboratory assessment for measuring peNDF for feeds using PSPS techniques.

Table 3. The effect of particle size of forage on chewing activity of cow[*]

Feed and particle size	NDF	Total chewing activity	
	% of DM	min/kg DM	min/kg NDF
Alfalfa hay			
Long	54	72	134
Chopped (3.8 cm)	54	59	109
Bermudagrass hay			
Long	72	108	149
Chopped (3.8 cm)	72	85	118
Alfalfa hay			
Long	53	62	117
chopped (3.8 cm)	53	44	84
Oat straw			
Long	84[1]	163	194
Ground	75[1]	84	113
Ryegrass			
Long	65[1]	90	139
Finely ground (1.2 cm)	64[1]	19	29
Corn silage			
1.9 cm TLC[2]	68	66	97
1.3 cm TLC	62	60	96
0.6 cm TLC	60	40	66
Alfalfa hay			
2.5 cm TLC	55	52	95
0.5 cm TLC	45	30	66

[*] Adopted from Mertens, 1997.

[1] NDF calculated from crude fiber concentration.

[2] Theoretical length of cut.

5.3. Optimum Physically Effective NDF in Terms of Rumen pH

Zebeli et al. (2006) reported that increasing the dietary peNDF content in dairy cows ration increases rumen pH quadratically. According to their meta-analysis the peNDF estimates rumen pH with $R^2 = 0.67$ and a root mean square error of 0.137 pH units. Mertens (1997) also reported a quadratic relationship ($R^2 = 0.71$) between dietary peNDF and rumen pH. Pitt et al. (1996) used data from beef cattle, dairy cattle and sheep, and observed a quadratic relationship ($R^2 = 0.52$) between peNDF and rumen pH. The quadratic relationship means that with increasing peNDF content of the ration, the rumen pH does not increase indefinitely; rather it attains an asymptotic plateau. The mathematical asymptotic function revealed a plateau at a rumen pH of ~6.2, in response to about 30% dietary peNDF (Zebeli et al., 2010). A further increase in peNDF does not increase rumen pH.

According to Zebeli et al. (2006) an intake of peNDF of either 4.1 kg/d, or concentration of >19% of ration DM is needed to maintain a pH of 6.0 and normal milk fat content. Mertens (1997) suggested that the peNDF amount needed to maintain a rumen pH of 6.0 should be arranged ±1.0 to 2.0 units of a mean of 22%.

The peNDF system has been adopted by a number of ration balancing programs, including the Cornell Net Carbohydrate and Protein System and by the CPM-Dairy.

5.4. Physically Effective NDF in Terms of Rumination and Milk Fat Content

Among the systems proposed to estimate the minimum amount of fiber necessary in rations for lactating dairy cows, most have attempted to guide ration formulation by predicting the amount of chewing that various feedstuffs would generate or their relative effectiveness to maintain milk fat content (Mertens, 2002).

De Brabander et al. (2002) suggested that dairy cows should achieve between 59 and 72.8 min/kg of chewing time from forages to prevent ruminal disorders and milk fat depression. Tafaj et al. (2005) estimated that for dairy cows to achieve a chewing time of 74 min/kg of DM from long-chopped hay, diets should contain 28% NDF or 19% peNDF and 60% slowly degradable concentrate in the diet (Zebeli et al., 2006).

Mertens (1997) suggested that for cows to maintain 3.6% milk fat, they should achieve a chewing time of 36.1 min/kg of DM. Beauchemin et al. (1994) and Mertens (1997) concluded that effects of particle size on milk fat content were likely to be observed when NDF levels were lower than the minimum recommended requirement.

6. DIGESTIBILITY

The NDF contains an indigestible fraction (lignin) and potentially digestible fiber fractions, each of which degrades at its own rate. The extent of NDF digestion depends on the size of the indigestible fraction, and the competition between the rates of degradation and passage out of the rumen, of the potentially digestible fractions. The indigestible fraction is a major factor affecting the digestibility of NDF as it varies greatly and may exceed more than one half of the total NDF in the rumen.

Ruminal and total tract digestibility of the potentially digestible fractions of NDF is a function of rate of degradation and rate of passage of particulate matter out of the rumen. Rate of passage is dependent on feed particles size and its fragility (particle size reduction), particles buoyancy and rate of degradation of the potentially digestible fraction. There is a vast range in ruminal fiber degradability between and among forage and non-forage sources.

6.1. Factor Affecting NDF Degradability

Although NDF degradability changes during lactation and with ration composition, much of the variation in NDF degradability is caused by composition and structural differences among forage families, species and hybrids, and harvest maturity. As forage mature, the indigestible fraction of NDF increases and the rate of fermentation of the potentially digestible fraction decreases. As a result, fiber degradability generally decreases as forages mature within a cutting. In addition, environmental factors such as temperature, soil moisture and fertilization may affect the changes in fiber degradability during maturity. Particle buoyancy in the rumen can also affect NDF degradability.

When particles are actively fermenting, they release carbon dioxide and methane gas that makes the particles float in the rumen. Buoyant particles are often trapped in the fiber mat. As the fermentable NDF fraction decreases, less gas is produced and particles may become less buoyant and sink. Those particles that have low concentrations of fermentable fiber and ferment quickly, such as alfalfa, might pass from the rumen more quickly than particles that have more fermentable fiber and ferment slowly such as grasses.

Grasses generally have a higher potentially degradable fraction than legumes, but the degradation rate of grass is lower than legumes. At a higher retention time grasses give higher NDF degradability than legumes. Although grass NDF is generally more degradable than legume NDF, it may also be more filling and can reduce DMI because of higher retention time. In situation where DMI in more sensitive to rumen fill, legumes may allow higher intake than grasses, as legume NDF ferments faster and most likely sinks and passes from the rumen faster than grass NDF. At shorter ruminal retention times, legume may have greater dry matter degradability than grasses. Whereas grasses may have greater NDF degradability than legumes when fed to cows with longer ruminal retention times, such as during late lactation and dry period. Dry matter intake in high producing dairy cows is usually limited by physical fill during early lactation. Offering NDF sources that degrade and pass from the rumen more quickly may increase the energy intake.

6.2. Lignin and Fiber Degradability

Lignin is an indigestible fraction of plant cell walls that stiffen the plant and prevent lodging. The lignin content of plant cell walls has long been regarded as the major barrier for microbial fermentation of fiber, and a negative correlation between lignin content and NDF degradability has been reported for grasses, silage maize and legumes. The indigestible NDF content of forages is estimated as 2.4 × lignin content (Lanzas et al., 2007). Forages with lower lignin content in cell walls (i.e., harvested early in the growing season and genetically modified for lower lignin content) degrades rapidly in the rumen and support high in DMI.

The proportion of lignin in NDF is directly related to its digestibility and filling effects. Fiber that is less lignified clears from the rumen faster, allowing more space for the next meal. However, ruminal retention time of NDF from perennial grasses is generally longer than NDF from legumes despite being less lignified (Oba and Allen, 1999; Voelker and Allen, 2008). These finding shows that lignin content explains variation in NDF degradability within a forage type but not across different forages. From a series of systematic research studies, which aimed to explore the variation in NDF degradability in silage maize due to genotypes, growth conditions and harvest maturity, it was concluded that not only lignin content but also the cross linkage of lignin with fiber as well as secondary cell wall thickness explains most but not all the variation in NDF degradability (Khan et al., 2014). Lignin content is a function of forage type, and generally increases with increasing harvest maturity. In addition, plant secondary cell walls thickness increases with maturity, with a consequent decrease in their fragility. The stage of maturity at harvest has therefore a profound influence on fiber degradability within a forage type.

6.3. Increasing NDF Degradability

Increasing the NDF degradability through plant breeding is a challenging goal. Selection forage cultivars for lower lignin content have been shown to increase NDF degradability. For example an improvement in NDF degradability of 19% for early brown midrib cultivars and 14.9% for late brown midrib cultivars of maize compared to normal cultivars has been reported (Barrière et al., 2003). However, the lower lignin content of brown midrib cultivars reduces the physical effectiveness of the NDF. Moreover, the effects of brown midrib cultivars on the total tract (in vivo) NDF digestibility are equivocal (Bal et al., 2000; Barrière et al., 2003). This inconsistency could be, partly, related to the opposing effect of rapid degradation and rumen-passage. Thus the increased DMI of lower lignin cultivars often increases the level but not the efficiency of milk production (Khan et al., 2014). As lignin content and its bonding with the fiber determine NDF degradability in the rumen, the degradability of NDF can be enhanced by treating it with lignin degrading enzymes.

So for the results of enzyme treatment is not very promising. Alternatively, some species of white rot fungi also selectively degrades lignin and improve the feeding value of low quality feeds such as cereal straws considerably. Fungi that are used to produce mushrooms on lignocellulose complexes are adapted to these complex substrates. These fungi have a strategy to colonize and modify the substrate in such a way that (hemi)cellulose is available when fruitbodies are produced. They preferentially produce enzymes directed to degrade or modify lignin during the vegetative growth and switch the enzyme system towards degradation of (hemi)cellulose during fruiting. By stopping the process before fruiting results in organic substrate with less lignin (bonds) and less limitations to breakdown of the cell wall carbohydrates. Supplementation of certain live yeasts such as *Saccharomyces cerevisiae* has shown consistent positive results, although the effect may be indirect through pH control. *S. cerevisiae* stimulates cellulolytic bacteria, and increases its potential to digest fiber in the rumen (Newbold et al., 2006). The cellulolytic bacteria is benefited due to the ability of *S. cerevisiae* to prevent a decrease in rumen pH by decreasing lactic acid production and stimulating the utilization of lactic acid by some bacteria, oxygen scavenging and supply of growth factors (Jouany, 2006).

6.4. NDF Digestibility and Dairy Cow Performance

Grant et al. (1995) and Dado and Allen (1996) fed silages with similar NDF and CP contents but different NDF digestibility to lactating dairy cows and found high DMI and milk yield with silage containing high digestible NDF. Oba and Allen (1999) conducted meta-analysis on published data from 7 experiments, and estimated that an 8.4% unit difference in NDF digestibility increased the DMI by 1.4 kg and fat corrected milk (FCM) by 2.1 kg. They further computed that a 1% unit increase in NDF digestibility measured *in vitro* or *in situ* can increase the DMI by of 0.17 kg and FCM by 0.25 kg. According to a more recent meta-analysis of Mertens (2006) a 1% unit increase in NDF digestibility can increase the DMI by of 0.097 kg and FCM by 0.14 kg. These findings show that dairy cows performance are improved when fed with more digestible NDF forages.

6.5. NDF Digestibility Measurement

Fiber digestibility is best determined by measuring the NDF digestibility during an *in vitro* fermentation. The NRC suggested that digestibility of NDF can be measured after 48 h incubation in buffered-rumen fluid according to the procedure of Tilley Terry (1963). However, other studies suggested that the 30 h incubation is much more sensitive in terms of rumen retention time and rumen turnover kinetics of lactating cows (Sniffen, 2010). The 30 h measurement is also sensitive to DMI and prediction of the dairy cow performance. Currently the system provides an endpoint value for NDF digestibility. As with other *in vitro* procedures there are several factors which could affect NDF digestibility. These include the dilution of the rumen fluid, type of buffer used, particle size of the sample and type of the diet fed to donor cow. Moreover, the *in vitro* procedure is using a dry, ground sample, which can decrease the difference in digestibility between samples or result in higher digestibility than unground wet samples.

7. DRY MATTER INTAKE

Fiber content and its digestibility is the primary regulator of DMI in dairy cows. From a meta analysis of 17 studies Mertens (2006) reported that ration NDF content has two times greater impact on DMI than NDF digestibility.

Similarly, the NDF content has three times greater impact on FCM yield than NDF digestibility. The greater impact of NDF content on DMI is related to the fact that fiber is the least digestible (40-70%) component of dairy ration, whereas non-fiber components (i.e., 100--NDF) have typically higher (> 90%) digestibility (Mertens, 1997).

These findings suggest that it is most important to formulate dairy ration for a recommended NDF content.

Once the ration is balanced for an optimal NDF content, then focus should be given to increase the NDF digestibility of the forages to improve DMI.

However, it is difficult to compensate for a higher NDF content in the ration with an improved NDF digestibility.

7.1. Mechanisms of Dry Matter Intake Regulations

The DMI of dairy cows, particularly of those with high milk yield, is regulated by physical fill under most dietary regimes. However, when the NDF content of dairy ration is very low, the DMI is regulated according to animal energy requirements. At a lower NDF content, intake is reduced because the diet is high in energy and animals reduce intake to match its energy demand. The extent to which this occurs in the range of diet NDF typically fed to dairy cattle appears to be small. As the NDF content of dairy ration increases, the DMI also increases because the ration is less dense in energy and more feed is required to meet the energy demand. At some point, the ration becomes so bulky that intake is limited by fill. These two mechanisms of intake regulation indicate that intake can increase, remain constant or decrease with changes in ration NDF content.

7.2. Intake Regulation by Physical Fill

The extent to which DMI of dairy cows is regulated by distension of reticulorumen is strongly dependent on the animal's energy requirement and the filling effect of the diet consumed. The DMI reduces with increasing filling effect of diet only when cows are in negative or slightly positive energy balance. It is expected that changing forage NDF content of the diet has more pronounced effect on DMI and milk yield of high producing cows as compared to low producing cows. In a study where two diets with different forage to concentrate ratio (24.3 *vs*. 30.7 % NDF) were fed to dairy cows producing different quantities of milk (Allen, 2010). With the higher NDF content the DMI and FCM decreased by ~4.5 and ~2.2 kg/d in high producing (> 40 kg FCM/d) cows. However, in the low producing (< 40 kg FCM/d) cows no differences in DMI and FCM was observed for the two diets. Similarly, Oba and Allen, (1999) compared the effect of feeding brown midrib and normal corn silage on DMI and milk yield of high (~55 kg/d) and low (~29.3 kg/d) producing dairy cows. The two silages had similar contents of DM and NDF, but *in vitro* NDF degradability (30 h) was nearly 25% (10 units) higher for the low-lignin brown midrib corn silage. The lower producing cows had similar DMI and FCM for the two silages, whereas feeding of brown midrib silages increase DMI and FCM by ~3.9 and ~8 kg/d in the high producing cows. These findings demonstrate that high producing dairy cows should be fed diets with lower filling effect to maximize feed intake.

7.3. Filling Effect of Various NDF Sources

Increasing diet NDF content by substituting non-forage fiber sources (NFFS) for concentrate feeds has shown little effect on DMI (Allen, 2000). The NFFS include byproduct feeds (i.e., cottonseeds, soyhulls, beet pulp, almond hulls, corn gluten feed, distiller's grains) with significant concentrations of NDF. Fiber in NFFS causes much less filling effect than forage NDF, because NFFS is less bulky initially, and over time in the rumen because it digests and passes from the rumen more quickly.

Forage NDF is less dense initially, digests more slowly, and is retained in the rumen longer than other diet components.

Retention time of forage NDF in the rumen is longer because of longer initial particle size and greater buoyancy in the rumen over time. The overall filling effect is a function of forage NDF content, forage particle size, fragility of forage NDF determined by forage type (legumes, perennial grasses, annual grasses), and NDF degradability within a forage family (Allen, 2000). As forages mature, the NDF fraction generally becomes more lignified and less fragile. Within a forage type, the degree to which NDF is lignified is directly related to the filling effects of the NDF.

Three is a significant interaction of NDF degradability and forage family on the filling effect of dairy cows. Although NDF degradability is often greater for grasses compared to legumes, the filling effect of legumes is less because of greater rate of particle size reduction (particles fragility) and rate of fermentation, which decreased retention time in the reticulrumen and resulted in less distension and greater DMI. On the other hand the greater potentially degradable NDF as a proportion of total NDF and slower rate of fermentation of the potentially degradable NDF in grasses, are expected to extend the length of time particles are buoyant, reduce rate of passage, and increase the filling effect of NDF over time (Allen, 1996). Compared to grass, corn silage has smaller particle size and greater particle size reduction and rumen passage rate (Khan et al., 2014). Similar DMI has been observed for comparisons of alfalfa and corn silage (Grant et al., 1995; Dhiman and Satter, 1997). These findings suggests that the greater filling effects of grass NDF compared to legume and corn silage NDF is a limitation to perennial grasses.

7.4. Forage Particle Size and DMI

Experiments that have evaluated effects of forage particle size have generally shown small effects on DMI (Allen, 2000). In a recent meta-analysis (Ferraretto and Shaver, 2012), an indirect comparison of 24 published studies and 106 treatment means of maize silages showed no significant influence of particle size on DMI and milk yield of dairy cows. In another literature review (Allen, 2000), only 3 of 20 comparisons, in which the same source of forage (hay or silage) was chopped at two or more lengths, have reported a significant effect of forage particle length on DMI. It is evident from literature data that large particle size can reduce DMI of dairy cows, when high proportions of forages are fed. Beauchemin et al. (1994) reported an interaction between forage particle size (5 *vs.* 10 mm theoretical length of cut) and percentage of forage (alfalfa silage) in the diet (35 *vs.* 65%). When forage content was increased from 35 to 65%, the DMI was reduced nearly 3 kg/d with the diet containing the long chopped alfalfa silage, but less than 0.5 kg/d with the diet containing the short chopped forage. Tafaj et al. (2001) reported that reducing dietary hay particle size from 28.7 to 9.2 mm increased DMI by 13% only in a high-forage (~87% in DM) diet, but when a high-concentrate diet (>40% in DM) was fed no differences were observed in the DMI of sheep.

7.5. Importance of Maintaining Ruminal Fill

Ruminal distention limits DMI in high producing dairy cows during early lactation. However, it has little effect on DMI during the transition period. Formulating diets to maintain rumen fill with ingredients that are retained in the rumen longer, and have moderate rates of fermentation and high ruminal digestibility will likely benefit transition cows several ways.

These include the supply of consistent energy when feed intake decreases at calving, which will ultimately minimize the risk of metabolic disorders, mastitis and infectious disease. Glucose demand of fresh cows is high when glucose utilization for milk production outpaces gluconeogenesis by the liver. While cows require diets with adequate glucose precursors (i.e., starch from grains), it is important to also maintain rumen fill. This will help maintain plasma glucose and prevent even more rapid mobilization of body reserves compared to when diets are formulated with ingredients that disappear from the rumen quickly. Moreover, buffering capacity is directly related to the amount of digesta in the rumen. Therefore, diets formulated with ingredients that increase the amount of digesta in the rumen will have greater buffering capacity and will maintain buffer capacity longer, when DMI decreases. Diets formulated with ingredients that maintain digesta in the rumen longer when feed intake decreases will likely decrease risk of rumen acidosis and abomasal displacement.

On the other hand, during mid and late lactation an adequate amount of fiber is required in the diet to partition energy towards milk production. Energy partitioning between milk production and body condition varies as physiological state changes during lactation. During early lactation, more energy is portioned to milk production. After the peak lactation, insulin concentration and sensitivity of tissues increase and energy is increasingly partitioned to body condition, sometimes at the expense of milk yield. High-starch diets can increase milk yield of high producing cows during early lactation, however, they result in excessive gain in body condition as milk yield declines. For example during late lactation feeding of a 69% forage diet (0% corn grain) containing brown midrib corn silage increased energy partitioning to milk, decreased body weight gain without any significant changes in milk yield compared to a 40% forage diet (29 % corn grain) containing control corn silage (Allen, 2010). Similarly, substituting beet pulp for high-moisture corn up to 12% of diet DM decreased body condition score of late lactating cows without decreasing milk and milk fat yields (Voelker and Allen, 2003). A recent experiment conducted with cows in the last 2 months of lactation also showed that substitution of beet pulp for barley grain linearly decreased body condition score and maintained milk yield (Mahjoubi et al., 2009).

8. Fiber Characteristics and Methane Production

Agriculture contributes to the anthropogenic greenhouse gas emissions of carbon dioxide (CO_2), methane (CH_4) and nitrous oxide with about 21-25, 60 and 65-80% respectively (Moss et al., 2000). Methane is one of the most important greenhouse gases and is released into the atmosphere both by natural and anthropogenic sources (biomass, ruminants, etc.). The contribution to the CH_4 emission of monogastric animals is very low compared with the ruminants. Emissions from ruminant livestock are approximately 250 and 500 litre of CH_4/ day. When these CH_4 emissions are applied to the number of cattle in the world, the total emissions from cattle is equivalent to about 15% of global CH_4 (Johnson et al., 1995). Concerning ruminants, CH_4 is formed during the fermentation of the fiber in the rumen and the amount produced depends on the quality and quantity of the forages.

Feeding legumes compared to grasses tends to reduce CH_4, but this relationship is also influenced by the maturity of the forage when it is fed to the animals.

With the advance of the growing season, the fibre content increases in the growing plant, whereas the soluble carbohydrates decrease. Therefore forages harvested in an early development stage usually have a higher digestibility and energy content. Woodward et al. (2004) concluded that CH_4 emissions per mega joule in gross energy decreases when the digestibility of the feed increases. Moreover, legumes produce less CH_4 because they have lower NDF content and pass more quickly through the rumen. Methane production can be decreased by grinding and pelleting of forages, due to the decrease of the retention time compared with forages coarsely chopped.

Furthermore, it has been demonstrated that the ratio between propionic and acetic acid has a higher impact on CH_4 production. Roughage diets high in cellulose lead to volatile fatty acids with a very high proportion of acetic acid while diets with a high proportion of concentrates (starches) give a large amount of propionic acid and are conducive to reducing ruminal CH_4 production.

Also, selecting forages and concentrates high in non fiber carbohydrates may reduce CH_4 emissions. NDF is heterogeneous concerning its chemical composition, digestibility, and potential to produce CH_4. For example the highly digestible NDF in distillers' by-products produces half to one-third of the CH_4 per kilogram of DM digested *in vitro* compared with forages with similar DM digestibilities. It has been reported that digested hemicellulose produces only 37% CH4 relative to digested cellulose. Forage type also influences CH_4 production. Tropical grasses (C4) tend to be less digestible than temperate (C3) grasses due to their higher NDF content and greater lignifications, and produce more CH_4 per unit of intake. In contrast, tropical legumes are significantly less digestible and produce less CH_4 per unit of intake than temperate legumes (Archimède et al., 2011).

REFERENCES

Allen, M. S. 1995. Fiber requirements: Finding an optimum can be confusing. *Feedstuffs* 67: 13-16.

Allen, M. S. 1996. Physical constraints on voluntary intake of forage by ruminants. *J. Anim. Sci.* 74: 3063-3075.

Allen, M. S. 1997. Relationship between fermentation acid production in the rumen and the requirement for physically effective fiber. *J. Dairy Sci.* 80: 1447-1462.

Allen, M. S. 2000. Effects of diet on short-term regulation of feed intake by lactating dairy cattle. *J. Dairy Sci.* 83: 1598-1624.

Allen, M. S. 2010. Feed intake regulation and cell wall digestion characteristics. In: *International symposium on the role of plant cell walls in dairy cow nutrition and health,* pp. 17-20. Wageningen, Gelderland, The Netherlands.

Aman, P., Hesselman, K. 1985. An enzyme method for analysis of total mixed linkage beta glucans in cereal grains. *J. Cereal Sci.* 3: 231-237.

Archimède, H., Eugène, M., Marie Magdeleine, C., Boval, M., Martin, C., Morgavi, D. P., Lecomte, P., and Doreau, M., (2011). Comparison of methane production between C3 and C4 grasses and legumes. *Anim. Feed Sci. Technol.*, 166-167. p. 59-64.

Bal, M. A., Shaver, R. D., Al-Jobeile H., Coors, J. G., Lauer, J. G. 2000 Corn silage hybrid effects on intake, digestion, and milk production by dairy cows. *J. Dairy Sci.* 83: 2849-2858.

Barrière, Y., Guillet, C., Goffner, D., Pichon, M. 2003. Genetic variation and breeding strategies for improved cell wall digestibility in annual forage crops: a review. *Anim. Res.* 52: 193-228.

Beauchemin, K. A., Farr, B. I., Rode L. M., Schaalje, G. B. 1994. Effects of alfalfa chop length and supplementary long hay on chewing and milk production of dairy cows. *J. Dairy Sci.* 77: 1326-1339.

Chen, L., Zhang, X., Yu, P. 2014. Correlating Molecular Spectroscopy and Molecular Chemometrics to Explore Carbohydrate Functional Groups and Utilization of Co-products from Bio-Fuel and Bio-Brewing Processing. *J. Agric. Food Chem.* 62: 5108-5117.

Dado, R. G., Allen, M. S. 1996. Enhanced intake and production of cows offered ensiled alfalfa with higher neutral detergent fiber digestibility. *J. Dairy Sci.* 79: 418-428.

De Brabander, D. L., De Boever, J. L., Vanacker, J. M., Boucque, C. V., Botterman, S. M. 1999. Evaluation of physical structure in dairy cattle nutrition. In: *Recent Advances in Animal Nutrition,* P. C., Wiseman, J. (Ed.), pp. 111-145. Nottingham University Press, Nottingham, UK.

De Brabander, D. L., De Boever, J. L., Vanacker, J. M., Geerts, N. E. 2002. Evaluation and effects of physical structure in dairy cattle nutrition. In: *Recent developments and perspectives in bovine medicine,* M. Kaske, H. Scholz, M. Höltershinken (Ed.), pp. 182-197. Proceeding of XXII World Buiatrics Congress, Hanover, Germany.

Dhiman, T. R., Satter, L. D. 1997. Yield response of dairy cows fed different proportions of alfalfa silage and corn silage. *J. Dairy Sci.* 80: 2069-2082.

Einarson, M. S., Plaizier, J. C., Wittenberg, K. M. 2004. Effects of barley silage chop length on productivity and rumen conditions of lactating dairy cows fed total mixed ration. *J. Dairy Sci.* 87: 2987-2996.

Ferraretto, L. F., Shaver, R. D. 2012. Meta-analysis: effect of corn silage harvest practices on intake, digestion, and milk production by dairy cows. *Prof. Anim. Sci.* 28: 141-149.

Grant, R. J., Haddad, S. G., Moore, K. J., Pedersen, J. F. 1995. Brown midrib sorghum silage for mid lactation dairy cows. *J. Dairy Sci.* 78: 1970-1980.

Henneberg, W. and F. Stohmann. (1859). Uber das erhaltungsfutter volljahrigen rindviehs. *J. Landwirtsch* 3:485-551.

Ishler, V., Varga, G. 2001. *Carbohydrate nutrition for lactating dairy cattle.* The Pennsilvania State University, code # DAS 01-29, pp. 1-11.

Johnson, K. A. and D. E. Johnson. (1995). Methane emissions from cattle. *J. Anim. Sci.* 73: 2483-2492.

Jonker, A., Gruber, M. Y., Wang, Y., Coulman, B., McKinnon, J. J., Christensen, J. J., Yu, P. 2012. Foam Stability of Leaves from Anthocyanidin-Accumulating Lc-Alfalfa and Relation to Molecular Structures Detected by FTIR Vibration Spectroscopy. *Grass Forage Sci.* 67: 369-381.

Jouany, J. P. 2006. Optimizing rumen functions in the close-up transition period and early lactation to drive dry matter intake and energy balance in cows. *Anim. Reprod. Sci.* 96: 250-264.

Khan, N. A., Yu, P., Ali, M., Cone, J. W., Hendriks, W. H. 2014. Nutritive value of maize silage in relation to dairy cow performance and milk quality. *J. Sci. Food Agric.* In press: DOI, 10.1002/jsfa.6703.

Kononoff, P. J., Heinrichs, A. J. 2003. The effect of reducing alfalfa haylage particle size on cows in early lactation. *J. Dairy Sci.* 86: 1445-1457.

Lammers, B. P., Buckmaster, D. R., Heinrichs, A. J. 1996. A simple method for the analysis of particle sizes of forage and total mixed rations. *J. Dairy Sci.* 79: 922-928.

Lanzas, C., Sniffen, C. J., Seo, S., Tedeschi, L. O., Fox, D. G. 2007. A revised CNCPS feed carbohydrate fractionation scheme for formulating rations for ruminants. *Anim. Feed Sci. Technol.* 136: 167-190.

Lowry, J. B., Conlan, L. L., Schlink, A. C., McSweeney, C. S. 1994. Acid detergent dispersible lignin in tropical grasses. *J. Sci. Food Agric*. 65: 41-49.

Mahjoubi, E., Amanlou, H., Zahmatkesh, D., Ghelich, Khan, M., Aghaziarati, N. 2009. Use of beet pulp as a replacement for barley grain to manage body condition score in over-conditioned late lactation cows. *Anim. Feed Sci. Technol*. 153: 60-67.

Mertens, D. R. 1997. Creating a system for meeting the fiber requirements of dairy cows. *J. Dairy Sci.* 80: 1463-1481.

Mertens, D. R. 2002. Physical and chemical characteristics of fiber affecting dairy cow performance. In: *Proceeding of Cornell Nutrition Conference on Feed Manufacturing*, pp. 125-144. Cornell University, Ithaca, NY, US.

Mertens, D. R. 2006. Do we need to consider ndf digestibility in the formulation of ruminant diets? In: *27th Western Nutrition Conference*, pp. 75-98. Winnipeg, Manitoba, Canada.

Mertens, D. R. 2009. Impact of NDF content and digestibility on dairy cow performance. In: *WCDS Advances in Dairy Technology.* volume 21: 191-201.

Moore, K. J., Hatfield, R. D. 1994. Carbohydrates and forage quality. In: Fahey, G. C., Jr., Collins, M. C., Mertens, D. R., Moser, L. E., (Ed.) *Forage quality, evaluation, and utilization,* pp. 229-280. ASA, CSSA and SSA, Madison, WI, US.

Moss, A. R., J. Jouany and J. Newbold. (2000). Methane production by ruminants: Its contribution to global warming. *Ann. Zootech*. 49, 231-253.

Newbold, C. J., Olvera-Ramirez, A. 2006. The use of yeast-based probiotics to meet new challenges in ruminant production. *J. Anim. Sci.* 84 (Suppl. 1), 425.

NRC, (2001). *Nutrient requirements of dairy cattle* (7th rev. edn.). National Research Council, National Academy of Science, Washington, DC. US.

Oba, M., Allen, M. S. 1999. Evaluation of the importance of the digestibility of neutral detergent fiber from forage: effects on dry matter intake and milk yield of dairy cows. *J. Dairy Sci.* 82: 589-596.

Pitt, R. E., Van Kessel, J. S., Fox, D. G., Pell, A. N., Barry, M. C., Van Soest, P. J. 1996. Prediction of ruminal volatile fatty acids and pH within the net carbohydrate and protein system. *J. Dairy Sci.* 74: 226.

Sniffen, C. J. 2010. Effect of NDF digestibility on diet formulation and animal performance. In: *International symposium on the "Role of plant cell walls in dairy cow nutrition and health"*, pp. 31-33. Wageningen, Gelderland, The Netherlands.

Tilley, J. M. A., Terry, R. A. 1963. A two-stage technique for the in vitro digestion of forage crops. *J. Brit. Grassl. Soc.* 18, 104-111.

Tafaj, M., Steingass, H., Drochner, W. 2001. Influence of hay particle size at different concentrate and feeding levels on digestive processes and feed intake in ruminants. 2. Passage, digestibility and feed intake. *Arch. Anim. Nutr.* 54, 243-259.

Tafaj, M., Maulbetsch, A., Zebeli, Q., Steingass, H., Drochner, W. 2005. Effects of physically effective fiber concentration of diets consisting of hay and slowly degradable concentrate on chewing activity in mid lactation dairy cows under constant intake level. *Arch. Anim. Nutr.* 59: 313-324.

Van Soest, P. J. 1963. Use of detergents in the analysis of fibrous feeds. II. A rapid method for the determination of fiber and lignin. *J. Assoc. Off. Anal. Chem.* 46: 829-835.

Van Soest, P. J. (1994). *Nutritional ecology of the ruminant*, 2nd ed. Comstock, Cornell Univ. Press, Ithaca, NY, US.

Van Soest, P. J., Robertson, J. B., Lewis, B. A. 1991. Methods for dietary fiber, neutral-detergent fiber and nonstarch polysaccharides in relation to animal nutrition. *J. Dairy Sci.* 74: 3583-3597.

Voelker, J. A., Allen, M. S. 2003. Pelleted beet pulp substituted for high-moisture corn: 1. Effects on feed intake, chewing behavior, and milk production of lactating dairy cows. *J. Dairy Sci.* 86: 3542-3552.

Voelker Linton, J. A., Allen, M. S. 2008. Nutrient demand interacts with forage family to affect intake and digestion responses in dairy cows. *J. Dairy Sci.* 91:2694-2701.

Woodward, S. L., G. C. Waghorn and P. G. Laboyrie. (2004). Condensed tannins in birdsfoot trefoil (Lotus corniculatus) reduce methane emissions from dairy cows. *Proceeding of the New Zealand Society of Animal Production.* 64.

Yang, W. Z., Beauchemin, K. A. 2006. Physically effective fiber: method of determination and effects on chewing, ruminal acidosis, and digestion by dairy cows. *J. Dairy Sci.* 89, 2618-2633.

Yu, P., Gamage, I. H. Zhang, X. 2014. New Approaches and Recent Advances on Characterization of Chemical Functional Groups and Structures, Physiochemical Property and Nutritional Values in Feedstocks and By-Products: Advanced Spectroanlytical and Modeling Investigations. *Applied Spectroscopy Reviews.* 49:585-602 (DOI:10.1080/05704928.2013.879064).

Yu, P., Zhang, X. 2014. Book Chapter: Raman Microspectroscopy (RMMS) for Exploration of Feed Structure and Nutrition Interaction: Using Non-Invasive Techniques in Animal Nutrition, In: *Microscopy: Advances in Scientific Research and Education*, Microscopy Book Series Volume - Number 6: Vol. 2 ISBN (13): 978-84-942134-4-1; Editor: A. Méndez-Vilas; pp. 747-751. Published by Formatex Research Center, Spain.

Zebeli, Q., Mansmann, D., Steingass, H., Ametaj, B. N. 2010. Balancing diets for physically effective fibre and ruminally degradable starch: A key to lower the risk of sub-acute rumen acidosis and improve productivity of dairy cattle. *Livest Sci.,* 127:1-10.

Zebeli, Q., Tafaj, M., Junck, B., Drochner, W. 2005. Effect of hay particle size and concentrate level on ruminal mat characteristics in dairy cows. In: *Proceeding of the Society of Nutrition Physiology*, pp. 14: 120 (Abstr.).

Zebeli, Q., Tafaj, M., Steingass, H., Metzler, B., Drochner, W. 2006. Effects of physically effective fiber on digestive processes and milk fat content in early lactating dairy cows fed total mixed rations. *J. Dairy Sci.* 89: 651-668.

In: Dietary Fiber
Editor: Marvin E. Clemens

ISBN: 978-1-63463-655-1
© 2015 Nova Science Publishers, Inc.

Chapter 6

PHYSICOCHEMICAL PROPERTIES AND RHEOLOGICAL BEHAVIOR OF DIETARY FIBER CONCENTRATES OBTAINED FROM PEACH AND QUINCE

Marina De Escalada Pla[1,2], Eim Valeria[3], Roselló Carmen[3], Gerschenson Lía Noemí[1,2,4*] and Femenia Antoni[3,4]

[1]Department of Industry, School of Exact and Natural Sciences, Buenos Aires University, Argentina
[2]Member of the National Scientific and Technical Research Council (CONICET), Argentina
[3]Department of Chemistry, Universitat de les IllesBalears, Ctra. Palma de Mallorca, Spain
[4]These authors contributed equally to the manuscript

ABSTRACT

Dietary fiber is a common and important ingredient in food product development. Its presence in food is desirable not only due to nutritional benefits but also for their functional and technological properties. In the present work, the rheology of four fiber fractions was evaluated. Two of them were obtained from quince waste which was submitted to different isolation processes: one with an ethanol treatment prior to drying and the other with distilled water washing previous to drying. The other fiber fractions were prepared from fresh peach pulp or peel. Suspensions of the fractions in deionized water were studied through dynamic tests. Weak gels of similar mechanical spectra were obtained when 2% w/w of peach fiber or 10% w/w of quince fiber suspensions were prepared in aqueous medium. Carbohydrate characteristics, particle size distribution and polidispersity influenced the rheological behavior. Mineral content was found to contribute to fiber nutritional value. Special attention should be paid to the process

[*]Corresponding author.Departamento de Industrias, FCEN, UBA Ciudad Universitaria, (1428) Buenos Aires. Argentina Tel.: +541145763366; fax: +541145763366. E-mail address: lia@di.fcen.uba.ar (L. N. Gerschenson).

applied for the obtention of dietary fiber concentrates in order to assure their adequate functionality.

Keywords: Dietary fiber, quince, peach, dynamic rheometry, carbohydrate, mineral composition

1. INTRODUCTION

According to current recommendations (Food and Nutrition Board, 2001), the average daily requirement of dietary fiber (DF) surpasses 20 g per day for women andis 30 g per day for men. Most nutritionists and diet experts suggest that 20-30% of our daily fiber intake should come from soluble fiber (Elleuch et al., 2011). In the last years, consumer demand for healthier food products with good sensorial properties has increased. Consumers demand DF is a common and important ingredient of these healthy food products (Gómez et al., 2003). Since consumer concerns are related to both nutritional and sensory aspects, a continuous evaluation and modification of the products and ingredients becomes essential in order to meet with consumer expectations (DelloStaffolo et al., 2004).

DF is an interesting ingredient not only for its nutritional benefits but also for its technological properties (Schieber et al., 2001) such as the capacity of increasing water and/or oil retention, the emulsifying properties and/or the formation of gels. However, the percentage of DF that can be added to a food is limited because this addition may cause undesirable changes to the color and texture of foods (Elleuch et al., 2008). Eim et al.(2008) were able to add 3% of carrot DF to dry fermented sausage (sobrassada) without observing undesirable texture changes in the final product. DelloStaffolo et al. (DelloStaffolo, 2004) studied the influence of DF from apple, wheat, bamboo or inulin on the sensory and rheological properties of yogurt. The effect of the addition of oat, wheat, apple and inulin fibers on the rheological properties of ice cream was reported by Soukoulis et al. (2009). Grigelmo-Miguel et al. (1999) studied the rheology of peach DF suspensions observing a pesudoplastic behavior. Augusto et al. (2011) studied the effect of the addition of peach DF to peach juice and observed that the product behaved as a viscoelastic system. deEscaladaPla et al. (2013) reported the enhancement of bread texture due to the addition of butternut fiber (0.5 – 1.5% w/w) without affecting crumb color. The type, as well as the extent of functional effects is undoubtedly related to the fiber's origin, the insoluble to soluble fiber ratio and the interactions with other food components (Soukoulis et al., 2009). Processing may cause irreversible modifications to the cell wall polysaccharides, affecting their original structure, hence the importance of selecting a process which guarantees the maintenance or enhancement of the fiber´s physical and functional properties.

The effect of the isolation procedure on the characteristics of DF obtained from quince and peach were reported previously (de EscaladaPla et al., 2010, 2012). Authors concluded in these publications that quince and peach were promising sources for obtaining fractions enriched in DF with the possibility of being used as food ingredients. The aim of this work was to deepen the characterization of these fractions through a collaborative work with the use of additional methodology. The characterization of mineral content of these fractions and of the dynamic rheological behavior of their aqueous suspensions was performed for the better evaluation of their technological application and health properties. Carbohydrate profiles, particle size distribution and polidispersity were also studied for a better understanding of the rheological behavior.

2. Materials and Methods

2.1. Fiber Fractions

The fiber fractions used were obtained for this research according to de EscaladaPla et al. (2010, 2012). Briefly, fiber fractions from quince (*Cydoniaoblonga*) were obtained from industrial pressed waste consisting of peel, seeds and stem, which was provided by a jelly manufacturer (Taxonera S.A., Mendoza, Argentina). Samples of this waste were submitted to different treatments. In the case of ME fraction, 100 g of sample were mixed with 350 ml of 96%v/v ethanol and boiled for 30 min under stirring, filtered to eliminate the most of extracting liquids and then dried under air convection at 30°C during 24 h. In the case of MA fraction, 100 g of sample were mixed with 350 ml of distilled water at 35°C for 30 min under stirring, followed by the same procedure above indicated for ME. Fiber fractions from peach (*Prunuspersica*) pulp (P) and peel (C) were obtained from fresh peaches (variety Calred, San Pedro, Buenos Aires province, Argentina) following a method similar to the one used for ME but with a drying period of 7 hours.

2.2. Chemical Analysis

Deionized water (MilliQ™, USA) was used for all assays. Ethanol used was of USP grade. Chemicals were of analytical grade and, in general, provided by MERCK Argentina (Buenos Aires, Argentina) unless stated. D-galacturonic acid was provided by SIGMA-Aldrich (St Louis, MO).

Alcohol insoluble residue (AIR) was obtained by treating each fiber product with boiling ethanol (USP grade, 96% v/v), according to de EscaladaPla et al. (2007). Briefly, one hundred grams of product were mixed with 350 mL of 96% v/v-ethanol solution and boiled for 15 min under stirring. The residue obtained was then extracted: (a) with 350 mL of 80% v/v-ethanol solution under boiling, for 15 min; and (b) twice with 250 mL of 80% v/v-ethanol solution under boiling, for 15 min. The insoluble residue was separated and washed with 100 mL of 80% v/v- and 100 mL of 96% v/v-ethanol solutions. Between each ethanol treatment, the suspension was filtered and the solvent was discarded. The AIR of each fiber product was left overnight under lab hood to eliminate the remaining ethanol and, finally, frozen with liquid nitrogen and freeze dried. AIR determination was performed at least in duplicate. The water soluble fraction (WSF) was also extracted as indicated by Ng and Waldron (1997). Briefly, each sample (0.5 g) was stirred in deionized water (MilliQ™, USA) (50 ml) for 2 hours at 20ºC, then filtered through glass fiber pad, frozen with liquid nitrogen and freeze dried. WSF was determined as difference between the weight of sample and the weight of the dried water insoluble residue. Filtered WSF was used in the light dynamic scattering assay.

Carbohydrate analysis was performed according to Femenia et al. (1998a). Sugars were released from polysaccharides by acid hydrolysis. Samples (≈5 mg) were dispersed in 72%

(w/w) H_2SO_4 for 3 h, followed by dilution to 1 M, and hydrolysis at 100 °C for 2.5 h (Saeman et al., 1954). A second sample was hydrolyzed with only 1 M sulfuric acid (100 °C for 2.5 h) and the cellulose content was estimated by the difference in glucose obtained by Saeman hydrolysis (Saeman et al., 1954) and this milder hydrolysis method. Neutral sugars were derivatized as their alditol acetates and isothermally separated by GC (Selvendran et al., 1979) at 220 °C on a 3% OV225 Chromosorb WHP 100/120 mesh column. Uronic acids were colorimetrically determined (Filisetti-Cozzi and Carpita, 1991) using a sample hydrolyzed for 1 h at 100 °C in 1 M H_2SO_4. The values for carbohydrates given in this paper correspond to the average of duplicate determinations.

In order to evaluate the possible amount of pectic polysaccharides and hemicellulosic moieties present, the method proposed by Arnous and Meyer (2009) was employed. Briefly, on the basis of monosaccharide analysis after acid hydrolysis of fiber products, an iterative calculation method was applied for the quantitative allocation of plant cell wall monomers into relevant structural polysaccharide elements. Then, molar percents of mannans, xyloglucans and arabinans could be estimated and the sum of them was considered as hemicellulosic polysaccharides. Similarly, RG-I, RG-II, arabinogalactan and homogalacturonans were estimated and the sum of them was considered as pectic polysaccharides (Pornsak, 2003).

Degree of branching (DB) was estimated from the molar ratio (Gal + Ara) / Rha according to Ngouémazong et al. (2012). Briefly, as rhamnose constitutes the branching point of RGI backbone while both galactose and arabinose are the major side chain neutral sugars, DB was determined as the ratio of the sum of the molar amounts of side chain neutral sugars over the molar amount of rhamnose as follows:

DB= (galactose+arabinose) / rhamnose

Fourier transform infrared spectroscopy (FTIR) was performed on a Bruker IFS 66 instrument (BrukerOptik GmbH, Ettlingen, Germany) at a resolution of 3 cm^{-1} using a KBr disk containing approximately 2 mg of sample. The intensity of the single beam traversing each sample was normalized with respect to the intensity of the single beam of the corresponding background. Equivalent samples from different experimental runs gave the same spectra in all cases.

2.3. Mineral Analysis and Microstructure Observation

DF products were observed by environmental scanning electronic microscopy, using a microscope model FEI XL30 ESEM FEI (FEI, Eindhoven, The Netherlands) with BrukerXFlash 4010 EDS detector (Bruker Nano GmbH, Berlin, Germany). In order to concentrate cell wall minerals, the ash from the AIR of each fiber product was obtained (AOAC, 2006). Then, estimation of mineral content was carried out on AIR ashes, through the microanalysis system with spectroscopy by electron dispersion with a BrukerXFlash 4010 EDS detector. Ash preparations as well as microanalysis were performed at least in duplicate.

2.4. Dynamic Light Scattering (DLS)

Water soluble fractions (WSF) were studied by dynamic light scattering. Experiments were carried out in a Dynamic Laser Light Scattering instrument (Zetasizer Nano-Zs, Malvern Instruments, Worcestershire, UK) provided with a He-Ne laser (633 nm) and using a digital correlator (Model ZEN3600). Measurements were carried out at a fixed scattering angle of 173°. Solutions (~6 mg/ml) contained in a disposable polystyrene cuvette were measured ten times and the average value for each sample is reported.

To obtain size information in the present research there were used: (i) the cumulant analysis which fits a single exponential to the correlation function, to obtain the mean size (z-average diameter, $Z_{average}$), and (ii) the CONTIN analysis which fits a multiple exponential to the correlation function to obtain the percentile distribution of particle/aggregate sizes, providing a plot of the relative intensity of light scattered by particles of various size classes (intensity size distribution). Through Mie theory, the original intensity distribution could be converted into volume distribution (Camino et al., 2011).

2.5. Rheology. Dynamic Studies of Fiber Suspensions

For the rheological assays, suspensions of DF products were prepared with 2% w/w of peach fiber in deionized water (MilliQ®), in the case of P and C samples, and with 10% w/w of quince fiber in deionized water (MilliQ®) in the case of ME and MA samples. Systems were homogenized using an ultraturrax device (IKA® Works, Inc., Wilmington) during 1 min at 13000 rpm while the system was cooled in an ice bath in order to avoid over heating due to high speed stirring. Samples were kept at 20°C for 1 hour before measurements.

Oscillatory assays were performed using a controlled stress rheometer (PaarPhysica MCR 300, Anton Paar GMBH, Germany) equipped with parallel plates (PP 30/S-714). A gap size of one milimeter was set and data points were recorded after the steady state was reached. Amplitude sweeps were first performed in order to determine the linear viscoelastic range (LVR). Storage (G') and loss (G'') moduli as well as strain were recorded as a function of stress, at constant frequency of 0.1 Hz and temperature of 20°C. Constant strain amplitude of 0.5% was chosen for all systems, and frequency sweeps were performed to determine the mechanical spectra, as a minimum, in triplicate. G' and G'', as well as the tangent of the phase angle ($\tan \delta = G''/G'$) were obtained as a function of increasing angular frequency. Experimental data were modeled with a power law-type equation (Kim and You, 2006):

$$G' = A\,\omega^{n} \qquad (1)$$

$$G'' = B\,\omega^{q} \qquad (2)$$

where A, B, n and q are fitting parameters.

2.6. Statistical Analysis

The results are informed on the basis of their average and standard deviation (α: 0.05). Significant differences between samples were evaluated through ANOVA followed by pairwise multiple comparisons using Tukey's significant difference test (α: 0.05). The correlation between rheological parameters and composition was analyzed through the Pearson product moment coefficient (Rodgers and Nicewander, 1988).

Statistical analysis (Sokal and Rohlf, 1980) was performed using the Statgraphics Plus package (V 5.1, 2004, Rockville, MD, USA).

3. Results and Discussion

3.1. Carbohydrate Composition

The amount of AIR and WSF obtained from fractions C, P, MA and ME can be observed in Figure 1. The peach products showed higher ($p<0.05$) WSF recovery than those proceeding from quince waste. The AIR content did not show significant differences between samples, although a tendency to higher values for the P and C fractions could be observed.

Carbohydrate composition for the four products and for the AIR and WSF was determined and results are reported in Table 1. High non cellulosic total sugars (NCS) (more than 50% w/w) were observed in all samples analyzed with the exception of the MA product which presented a slight but significantly ($p<0.05$) lower value (Table 1). Around 65 to 73% of the NCS of each product corresponded to cell wall polysaccharides, as can be inferred from comparison with the NCS content in the respective AIR fractions. The presence of pectic polysaccharides was observed in the four products and could be inferred from the large amounts of uronic acids, galactose and arabinose, and from the occurrence of rhamnose (González-Centeno et al., 2010). Uronic content in peach DF (C and P) almost doubled that of MA and ME quince products. In addition, P presented the highest ($p<0.05$) content of rhamnose (Rha), fucose (Fuc) and arabinose (Ara). Rha and Ara are side chain substituents of the pectin structural unit: rhamnogalacturonan I (RGI) (Arnous and Metyer, 2009). According to Gonzalez-Centeno et al. (2010), the presence of xylose (Xyl), fucose (Fuc), mannose (Man) and non-cellulosic glucose may be indicative of the occurrence of hemicellulosic polysaccharides. To evaluate the amount of free glucose (Glc) in C, P, MA and ME products, the difference between the amount present in the fractions and in their AIR was estimated, because each fraction could have retained some free sugars despite the treatment applied before drying.

MA product presented the highest Xyl content while ME showed the highest non-cellulosic Glc value. The same difference was also observed when comparing the AIR of those fractions. Arnous and Meyer (2009) assumed a xyloglucan structure composed of a backbone made up of β-1,4-bonded glucose units with intermittent substitutions at C6 in the hemicelluloses of grape. Other authors proposed a linear β-1,4 xylose-glucose backbone structure in hemicelluloses of the skin of grapes with a molar xylose:glucose ratio of 1:0.1 (Igartuburu et al., 2009). MA and ME were produced from the same raw material but the former was submitted to water washing and the latter was ethanol treated and different polysaccharide fractions could have been lost during these treatments giving origin to the difference observed in the monosaccharide distribution found in MA and ME.

Table 1. Carbohydrate composition from C, P, MA and ME products assayed and their respective alcohol insoluble residue (AIR) and water soluble fraction (WSF)

	C	P	MA	ME
Fiber product				
Rhamnose	10.74 ± 0.03^{a}	13.33 ± 0.08^{b}	9.0 ± 0.6^{c}	$9.84 \pm 0.06^{a,c}$
Fucose	5.2 ± 0.3^{a}	7.3 ± 0.3^{b}	3.6 ± 0.5^{c}	3.59 ± 0.05^{c}
Arabinose	92 ± 1^{a}	113 ± 2^{b}	52.0 ± 0.3^{c}	66 ± 4^{d}
Xylose	$40.6 \pm 0.6^{a,c}$	34 ± 3^{a}	79 ± 5^{b}	55 ± 5^{c}
Mannose	18 ± 2^{a}	18 ± 2^{a}	9.20 ± 0.03^{b}	11.8 ± 0.5^{b}
Galactose	$42 \pm 8^{a,b}$	$59 \pm 4^{a,c}$	38.0 ± 0.9^{b}	$47.0 \pm 0.4^{b,c}$
Glucose	106 ± 2^{a}	$122 \pm 6^{a,b}$	125 ± 4^{b}	182 ± 2^{c}
Uronics	200 ± 20^{a}	240 ± 20^{a}	107 ± 7^{b}	134 ± 9^{b}
Total sugars	$510 \pm 30^{a,b}$	600 ± 40^{a}	420 ± 20^{b}	$510 \pm 20^{a,b}$
Cellulose	$120 \pm 20^{a,b}$	155 ± 8^{a}	$120 \pm 10^{a,b}$	90 ± 10^{b}
AIR				
Rhamnose	$9.9 \pm 0.8^{a,b}$	12 ± 2^{a}	6.9 ± 0.9^{b}	$8.9 \pm 0.5^{a,b}$
Fucose	6 ± 1^{a}	8.07 ± 0.09^{a}	2.19 ± 0.08^{b}	3.2 ± 0.2^{b}
Arabinose	94 ± 2^{a}	120 ± 10^{a}	39 ± 4^{b}	59 ± 3^{b}
Xylose	$40 \pm 2^{a,c}$	$34.1 \pm 0.7^{a,c}$	74 ± 9^{b}	50 ± 3^{c}
Mannose	14.2 ± 0.9^{a}	10.1 ± 0.4^{b}	6.2 ± 0.8^{c}	$8 \pm 1^{b,c}$
Galactose	33.5 ± 0.2^{a}	$58 \pm 9^{b,c}$	27 ± 4^{a}	$40 \pm 1^{a,c}$
Glucose	44 ± 2^{a}	21 ± 2^{b}	58 ± 7^{a}	110 ± 3^{c}
Uronics	160 ± 10^{a}	240 ± 10^{b}	142 ± 7^{a}	174 ± 4^{a}
Total sugars	$400 \pm 20^{a,b}$	500 ± 30^{a}	360 ± 30^{b}	$450 \pm 20^{a,b}$
Cellulose	$150 \pm 20^{a,b}$	176 ± 8^{a}	$160 \pm 20^{a,b}$	100 ± 8^{b}
WSF				
Rhamnose	$6.3 \pm 0.7^{a,b}$	7.8 ± 0.3^{a}	$5.35 \pm 0.06^{b,c}$	$6.6 \pm 0.2^{a,c}$
Fucose	$1.4 \pm 0.7^{a,b}$	2.3 ± 0.2^{a}	n/d	n/d
Arabinose	56 ± 5^{a}	60.9 ± 0.9^{a}	28 ± 1^{b}	51 ± 1^{a}
Xylose	7.2 ± 0.9^{a}	6.5 ± 0.8^{a}	11.3 ± 0.2^{b}	12.5 ± 0.5^{b}
Mannose	15.3 ± 0.9^{a}	14 ± 2^{a}	17 ± 2^{a}	15.3 ± 0.5^{a}
Galactose	35 ± 5^{a}	37 ± 1^{a}	15 ± 2^{b}	28 ± 2^{a}
Glucose	$204 \pm 1^{a,c}$	184 ± 7^{a}	300 ± 20^{b}	236 ± 8^{c}
Uronics	349 ± 6^{a}	370 ± 20^{a}	113 ± 5^{b}	182 ± 6^{c}
Total sugars	670 ± 20^{a}	680 ± 30^{a}	490 ± 30^{b}	430 ± 20^{b}

Different letters express significant differences ($p<0.05$) between fractions.
C: dietary fiber fraction from peach peel.
P: dietary fiber fraction from peach pulp.
MA: dietary fiber fraction from quince waste with aqueous treatment.
ME: dietary fiber fraction from quince waste with ethanol treatment.
Fiber product composition:reported as µg of sugar / mg dried fiber product dry basis.
AIR composition: reported as µg of sugar / mg AIR dry basis.
WSFcomposition: reported as µg of sugar / mg WSF dry basis.

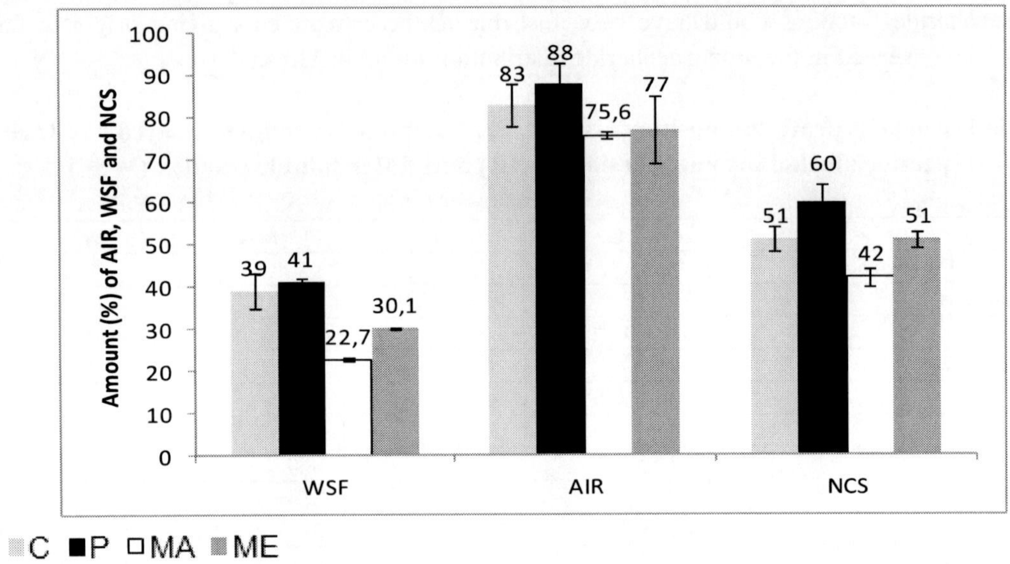

Figure 1. Amount (g/100 g dried sample) of alcohol insoluble residue (AIR), water soluble fraction (WSF) and non cellulosic carbohydrates (NCS) in the C: dietary fiber from peach peel; P: dietary fiber from peach pulp; MA: dietary fiber from quince waste obtained with aqueous treatment and, ME: dietary fiber from quince waste obtained with ethanol treatment.

The hemicellulosic and pectic polysaccharides calculated from monosaccharides according to Arnous and Meyer (2009) and the degree of branching (DB) are shown in Figure 2. It can be observed that fiber obtained from peach pulp (P) presented the highest pectin content ($p<0.05$) and its DB was slightly higher although the difference was not significant (Figure 2A). On the other hand, ethanol treatment previous to drying (ME) tended to reduce hemicellulosic (Figure 2A) and cellulosic (Table 1) contents in fiber products obtained from quince waste. This change in the polysaccharide distribution could also be corroborated through the FT-IR analysis discussed below (Section 3.2).

3.2. FT-IR Spectroscopy

Figure 3 shows FT-IR spectra of fiber products (Figure 3 A, B, C and D) and those obtained from their WSF (Figure 3 E, F, G and H). Bands between 1200 and 600 $cm^{-1}$are said to lie in the "fingerprint" region, because this part of the spectrum is unique for each particular compound, althoughindividual peaks cannot be assigned (McCann et al., 1992). The spectrum of fiber products coming from quince (MA and ME) showed a clearly different profile in this region when compared with those from peach (P and C). In addition, water (MA) or ethanol treatment (ME) seemed not to influence the profile (Figure 3 A and B). Bands observed at 1619 cm^{-1} correspond to the symmetrical stretching vibration of COO^- group (Manrique and Lajolo, 2002). These bands probably overlapped with amide-stretching bands (1640 cm^{-1}) of protein associated to the cell wall that may be present in fiber products (Femenia et al., 1998a, 1998b). The band that appears at about 1740 cm^{-1} can be assigned to C=O stretching vibration of methyl esterified carboxylic group (Manrique and Lajolo, 2002) and different absorbance intensities detected, reflect the different degree of esterification exhibited by pectic polysaccharides. Although no difference in intensity could be detected at 1740 cm^{-1} for MA and ME (Figure 3 A and B), a marked decrease of this signal was observed in the spectra of their WSF (Figure 3 E and F), being this trend more evident for the WSF of MA. Conversely, pectic polysaccharides with a high degree of methylation seemed to be present in the WSF of peach fiber (P and C) (Figure3 C and D). deEscaladaPla et al. (2010, 2013) reported high DM for DF from peach pulp and peel, and low DM for quince DF. In addition, it was observed a lower intensity in the "fingerprint" region corresponding to pectic polysaccharide bands (also with different shape), for the WSF of MA in comparison to the WSF of ME, confirming the difference observed in the polysaccharide distributions (Figure 2 B) probably caused by the treatment applied previous to drying, as discussed above.

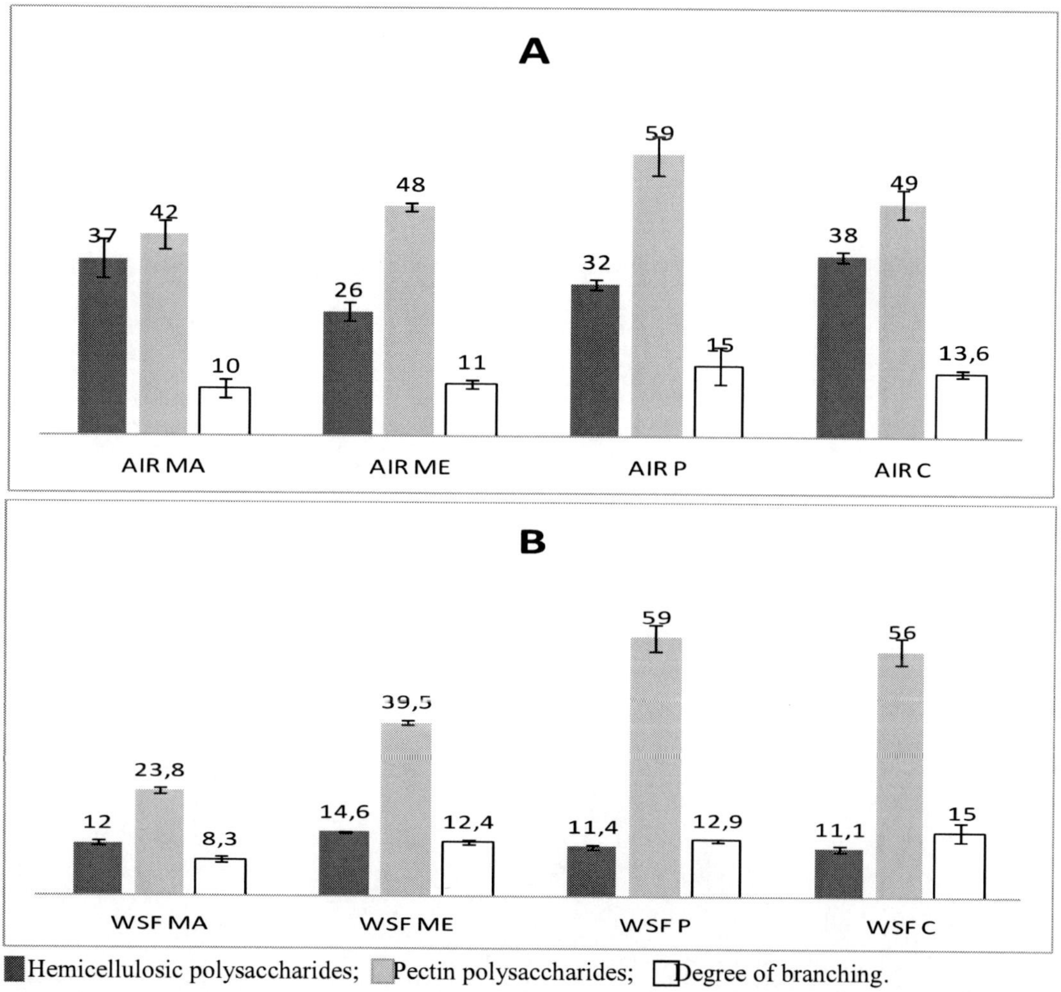

Figure 2. Polysaccharide content (percentual molar relation) and degree of branching for alcohol insoluble residue (AIR) of C: dietary fiber from peach peel; P: dietary fiber from peach pulp; MA: dietary fiber from quince waste obtained with aqueous treatment and ME: dietary fiber from quince waste obtained with ethanol treatment (Panel A) and for water soluble fraction (WSF) of C, P, MA and ME (Panel B).

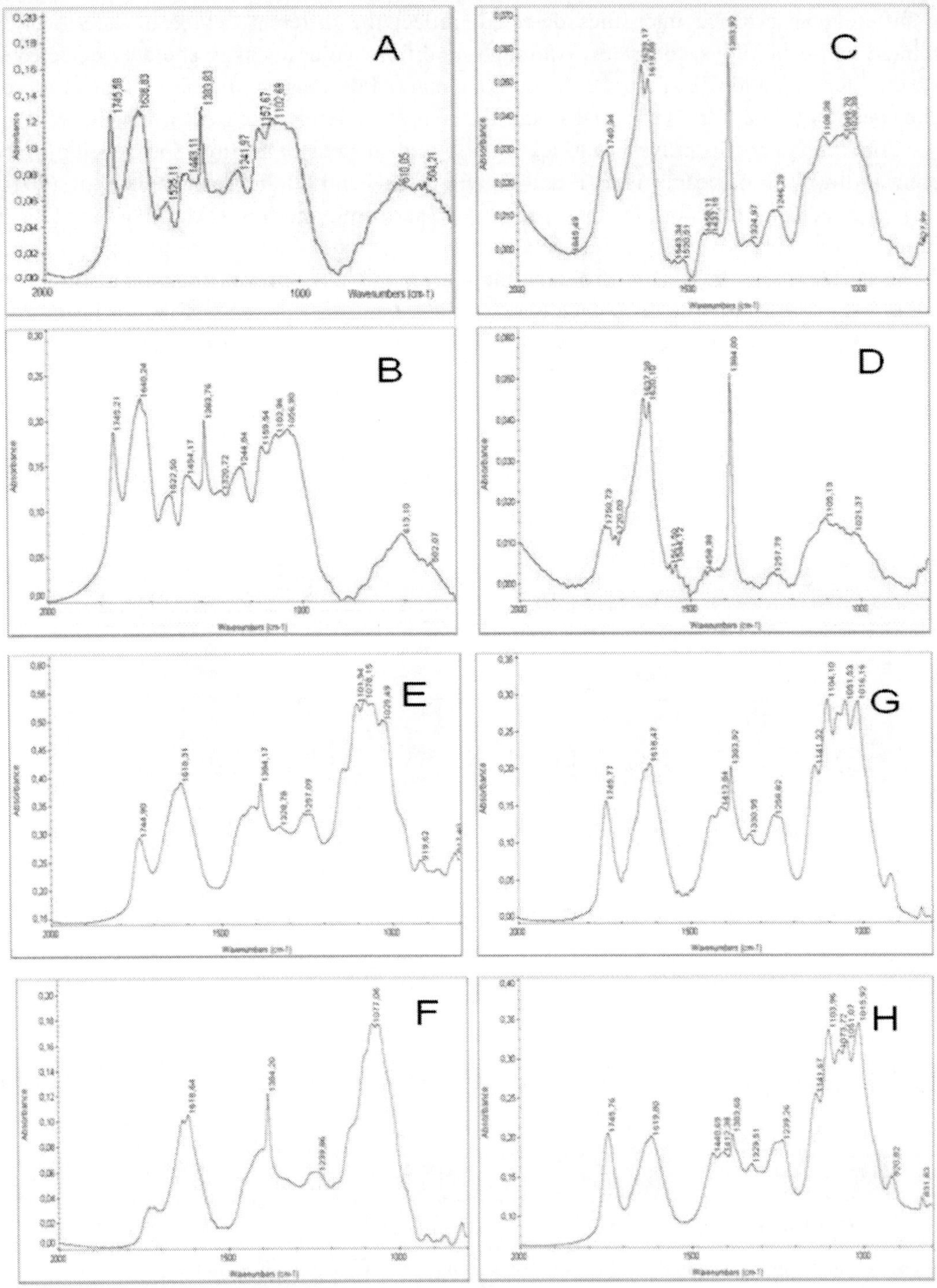

Figure 3. Fourier transform infrared spectroscopy (FTIR) spectra for dietary fiber from quince waste obtained with ethanol treatment, ME(Panel A);dietary fiber from quince waste obtained with aqueous treatment, MA (Panel B);dietary fiber from peach peel, C (Panel C);dietary fiber from peach pulp, P (Panel D); water soluble fraction (WSF) of ME (Panel E);WSF of MA (Panel F), WSF of C (Panel G) and WSF of P (Panel H).

3.3. Mineral Elements Associated with Cell Wall

The prevailing mineral elements that could be detected in the ashes of AIRs through energy-dispersive X-ray spectroscopy (RX-EDS) are reported in Table 2. Non significant differences could be observed between individual mineral elements of AIRs from the four fiber products but it is interesting to note that, in all cases, the Ca content was approximately 10 times greater than that of Na.

Ca, K, P and Mg were the four most abundant elements and their relative quantity is reported in Figure 4. Ca was the predominant element in AIR from C, MA and ME followed by K while a highest proportion of K was observed for AIR of sample P. Whilst high levels of Ca and Mg may be related to highest values of firmness, the high level of Na and K has a double effect because it might improve texture by reducing the electrostatic repulsion of acidic groups but it can also exert the opposite effect on texture due to the competition of Na and K with Ca (Van Buren, 1979). The interaction of monovalent cations with the carboxyl groups inhibits the ability of pectic polysaccharides to form cross-links, thus overall wall porosity may be increased in tissues coming from peach pulp (Femenia et al., 1998b).

It is important to state that 5 g of DF can provide around1.5-2% of the Ca dietary reference intake and 15-26% of the Fe dietary reference intake for males between 31 and 50 years, while this amount of fiber only provides around 0.1% of the adequate intake of Na and 0.2-0.4% of the adequate intake of K per day. It can be concluded that isolated DFs are a good source of iron (Food and Nutrition Board, 2005, 2011).

Table 2. Predominant mineral elements detectable in the ashes of alcohol insoluble residues (AIRs) through energy-dispersive X-ray spectroscopy (RX-EDS) expressed as μg mineral/mg of AIR

	AIR C	AIR P	AIR ME	AIR MA
Na	0.5 ± 0.2	0.28 ± 0.09	0.49 ± 0.07	0.4 ± 0.1
Mg	1.3 ± 0.3	1.1 ± 0.1	2.1 ± 0.2	1.66 ± 0.08
Al	0.11 ± 0.09	0.03 ± 0.01	n/d	n/d
Si	0.6 ± 0.2	0.05 ± 0.01	0.141 ± 0.006	0.16 ± 0.03
P	1.5 ⊥ 0.3	1.43 ± 0.05	2.2 ± 0.1	1.8 ± 0.3
S	0.7 ± 0.1	0.77 ± 0.03	0.9 ± 0.2	0.38 ± 0.03
K	4.6 ± 0.7	4.1 ± 0.4	4.5 ± 0.4	2.1 ± 0.4
Ca	5.3 ± 0.4	3.2 ± 0.2	5.5 ± 0.2	4.8 ± 0.9
Fe	0.5 ± 0.1	0.32 ± 0.07	0.33 ± 0.02	0.4 ± 0.2

AIR C: alcohol insoluble residue of dietary fiber fraction from peach peel.
AIR P: alcohol insoluble residue of dietary fiber fraction from peach pulp.
AIR ME:alcohol insoluble residue of dietary fiber fraction from quince waste with ethanol treatment.
AIR MA: alcohol insoluble residue of dietary fiber fraction from quince waste with aqueous treatment.

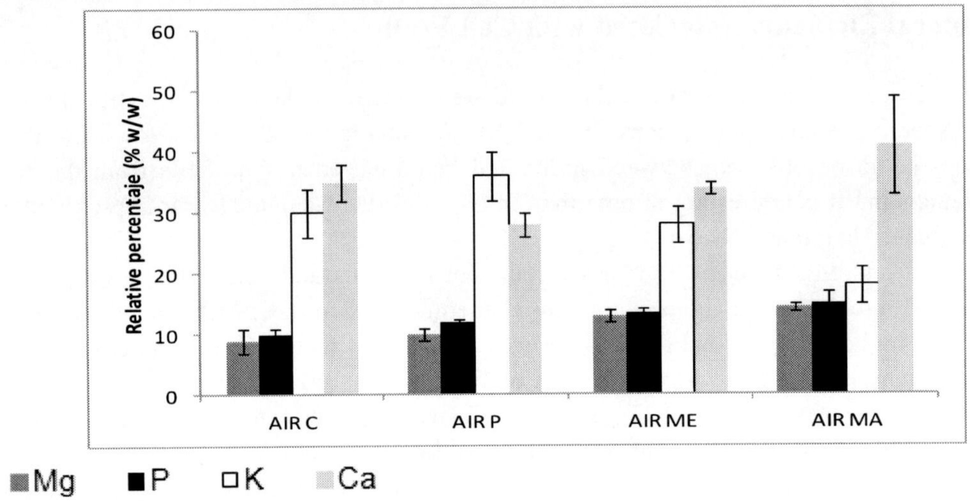

Figure 4. Relative percentage of predominant minerals in the alcohol insoluble residue (AIR) of: dietary fiber from peach peel (C), dietary fiber from peach pulp (P), dietary fiber from quince waste obtained with aqueous treatment (MA) and dietary fiber from quince waste obtained with ethanol treatment.(ME).

3.2. Particle Size Distribution of WSF Solutions

$Z_{average}$, which is the mean diameter of the ensemble of particles, was determined on the WSF of the different fractions. Values obtained in nanometers were: 1400 ± 200 for C, 800 ± 200 for P, 510 ± 80 for MA and 800 ± 100 for ME, MA being the fraction with the lowest values. This parameter is useful for comparison purposes it is notadequate for giving a complete description of the size distribution in polydisperse systems (Camino et al., 2009). The volume based size distributions are shown in Figure 5 where it can be observed that C fraction presented the highest mean hydraulic diameter followed by P and ME, while MA exhibited the lowest values. With the exception of C, the rest of the samples showed a multimodal distribution.

Non significant differences were observedon$Z_{average}$ when comparingP and ME samples, nevertheless the latter presented a bimodal distribution while P showed, in addition, a third small (≈ 20 nm) population (Figure 5). It must be stated that polysaccharide preparations are highly polydisperse (Murphy, 1997) and tend to form aggregates in aqueous media (Doublier and Launay, 1981) which can increase the elastic modulus (Funami et al., 2007). Possibly, the higher peaks observed could be attributed to aggregates.

3.3. Microstructural Observation

The functional properties of fibers are related to the structure-composition of constituent polysaccharides and are influenced by porosity and the particle size of the material (Femenia et al., 1997). Moreover, these properties depend on how these polymers are interconnected and arranged in space (Jarvis, 2011).

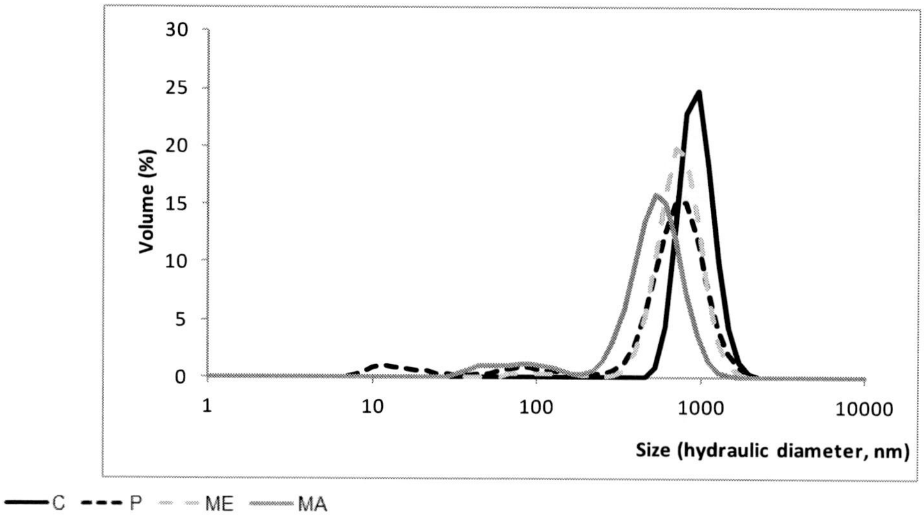

Figure 5. Volume based size distribution for the different water soluble fractions of dietary fiber obtained from: peach peel (C), peach pulp (P), quince waste obtained with aqueous treatment (MA) and quince waste obtained with ethanol treatment (ME).

In Figure 6, the roughness and porosity of the surface of the samples can clearly be observed. It is also interesting to note that some intact vascular structures typical of vegetable tissues could also be found on the samples obtained from peach pulp (Figure 6C) and peel (Figure 6D), These structures could not be observed on MA and ME sample surfaces because they were obtained from wastes from a previous industrial process which probably produced extensive damage. On the other hand, as microscopic observation of the product (Figures 6C and 6D) showed part of the original tissue structure, it could be concluded that the treatment applied for product isolation had assisted in its preservation. This is important considering that the nutritional value of cell walls depends on the extent to which they remain physically intact during the processing and the digestion (Jarvis, 2011). It is concluded that the raw material used, as well as the technological processes applied to isolate DF rich products, might condition the usefulness of the product isolated, and that it is important to select adequate processing conditions that allow optimizing fiber's functional properties.

3.4. Rheological Behavior. Dynamic Studies of Fiber Suspensions

Rheological behavior of fiber suspensions in deionized water was analyzed. Figure 7 shows mechanical spectra obtained for P fraction (Figure 7A), C fraction (Figure 7B), MA fraction (Figure 7C) and ME fraction (Figure 7D). It is important to note that it was not possible to evaluate the rheological behavior of MA and ME suspensions at concentrations lower than 10 % w/w because of their lack of stability.

Data obtained from aqueous systems through oscillatory testing in linear viscoelastic conditions show that the systems exhibited gel-like dynamic mechanical spectra; that is, the storage modulus G' predominated over the loss modulus G'' in the entire frequency range examined. However, the observed slight frequency dependence of the moduli and the relatively large value of tan δ (G''/G' > 0.1) were typical of the so-called weak gels (Ikeda and Nishinari, 2001; Alonso Mougán et al., 2002).

In the case of fraction P and ME, the difference between G' and G'' was of half an order of magnitude; in the case of C and MA it was lower. In all cases, the difference decreased with the increase in frequency. In the case of C and MA fractions, lower values of G' and G'' were observed and MA showed the higher values of tan δ revealing the greatest proportion of viscous behavior among these fractions. Although an important proportion of the fiber fraction was solubilized in water (Figure 1), another portion of insoluble fiber particles remained suspended in the viscous solution probably determining the weak gel behavior observed.

Table 3. Parameters obtained through the fitting of experimental data to power law model

	Storage Modulus (G')		Loss Modulus (G'')	
	A	n	B	q
P	160 ± 40^{a}	0.144 ± 0.002^{a}	26 ± 7^{a}	0.35 ± 0.02^{a}
C	69 ± 8^{b}	0.16 ± 0.01^{a}	11 ± 1^{b}	0.407 ± 0.009^{b}
ME	240 ± 20^{c}	0.088 ± 0.009^{b}	29 ± 3^{a}	$0.38 \pm 0.01^{a,b}$
MA	81.9 ± 0.6^{b}	0.084 ± 0.003^{b}	10.7 ± 0.5^{b}	0.48 ± 0.01^{c}

Different letters express significant differences (p<0.05) between fractions.
P: dietary fiber fraction from peach pulp.
C: dietary fiber fraction from peach peel.
ME: dietary fiber fraction from quince waste with ethanol treatment.
MA: dietary fiber fraction from quince waste with aqueous treatment.

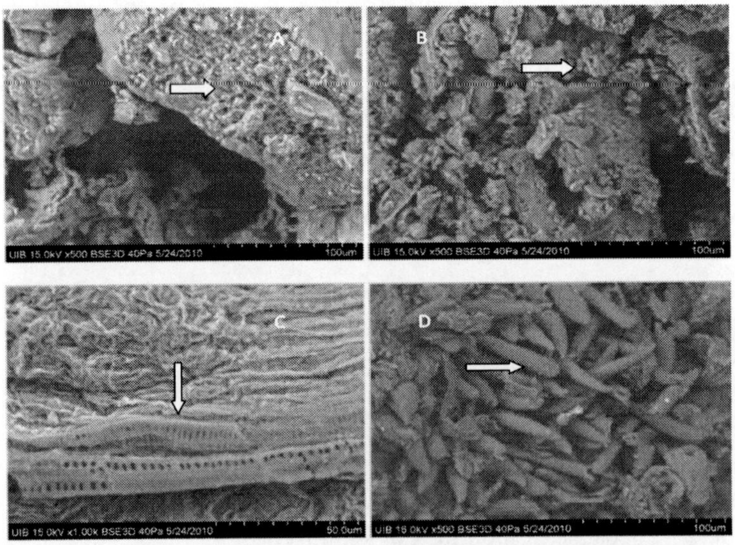

Figure 6. Electronic microscopy of product surfaces. Dietary fiber obtained from: quince waste with ethanol treatment ME (A), quince waste with aqueous treatment MA (B), peach pulp P (C) and peach peel C (D). For ME and MA, arrows show the presence of pores. For P and C, arrows point to vascular tissue. Magnification: for (A), (B) and (D), 500x; for (C), 1000x.

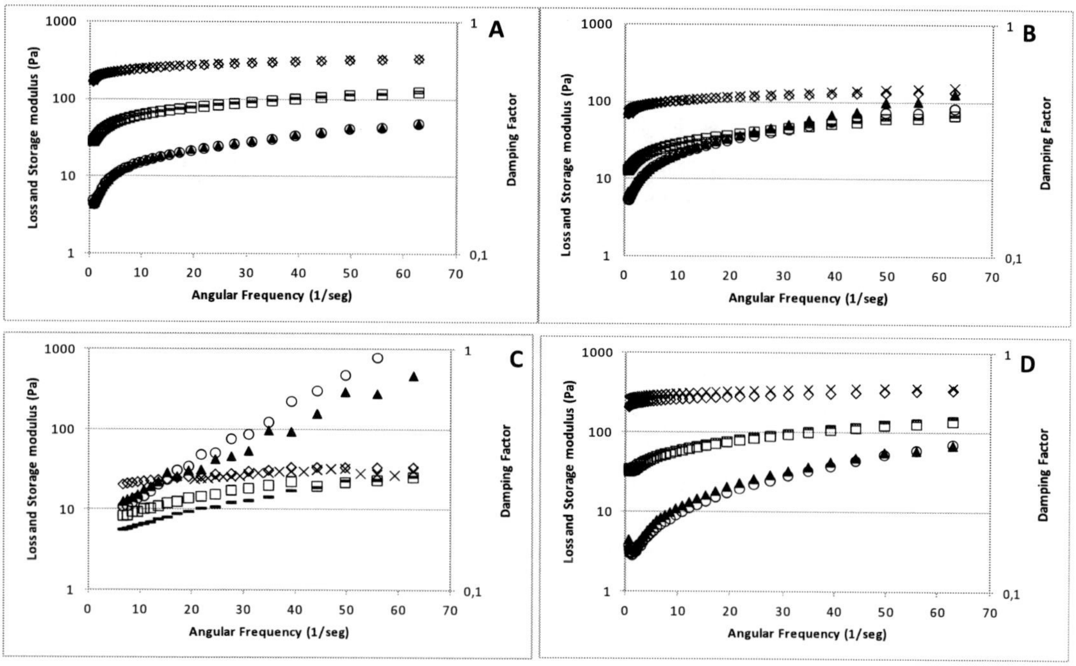

Figure 7. Dynamic rheometry for water suspensions of dietary fiber obtained from: A) peach pulp, P fraction (2%, w/v);B) peach peel, C fraction(2%, w/v); C) quince waste with aqueous treatment, MA fraction (10%, w/v)and D) quince waste with ethanoltreatment, ME fraction (10%, w/v). Two replicates are shown: ◊ and X represent Storage modulus (G'); □ and –represent Loss modulus (G''); ○ and ▲represent tan δ (damping factor).

Table 4. Pearson product moment correlation between the exponent n (power law equation describing the storage modulus, G') and the composition of the fractions. Inparentheses, the p-value corresponding to the statistical significance of the correlations. Between brackets, pairs of data used to calculate each coefficient

	AIR	DB	Hemicellulosic	NCS	Pectin^{-1}	Total Uronics	WSF^{-1}
n-exponent	-0,9858	0,5282	-0,9652	-0,9671	0,9690	-0,8096	0,9845
	[4]	[4]	[4]	[4]	[4]	[4]	[4]
	(0,0142)	*(0,4718)*	*(0,0348)*	*(0,0329)*	*(0,0310)*	*(0,1904)*	*(0,0155)*

p values lower than 0.05 indicate correlations significantly different from zero.

n: exponent obtained from fitting G'data to power law model ($G' = A\ \omega^n$).

AIR: alcohol insoluble residue content (g/100 g of water suspension).

DB: Degree of branching of water soluble polysaccharides.

Hemicellulosic: Molar content of hemicellulosic polysaccharides in water soluble fraction (moles/100 g water suspension).

NCS: mass content of non cellulosic sugars in water soluble fraction (g/100 g of water suspension).

Pectin: pectin polysaccharide content in water soluble fraction (g/100 g of water suspension).

Total uronics:uronic acidcontent in water soluble fraction (mg /100 g water suspension).

WSF: water soluble fraction content (g/100g water suspension).

The power law model satisfactorily fitted the experimental data, obtaining R^2 values in the range of 0.957-0.998 (Table 3). Higher q-exponents indicated that the loss modulus (G'') showed higher dependence on frequency than G' for all systems assayed. In addition, storage modulus of peach DF systems (P and C) was more dependent on frequency than that of quince fiber (MA and ME) suspensions. P system showed a more elastic behavior than C system (Figure 7), showing a higher "A" parameter and, simultaneously, the loss modulus (G'') for C system presented a slight but significant higher frequency dependence (higher "q") as can be observed in Table 3. Fissore, et al. (2012)characterized 2.00% w/v-aqueous systems of pectin enriched products extracted from red beet with calcium addition obtaining values of A: 9123 -19980; n: 0,069-0,083;B: 969-2302 andq: 0,097-0,158.

A 10% concentration of ME and MA was necessary to obtain G' values of the same order as those of fractions isolated from peach. The ME system showed a more elastic behavior than MA. These systems showed similar modulus values to those reported by Fissore et al. (2012) when working with gels obtained with 2% w/v red beet pectins and whole or skim milk. Values obtained for G' were higher than those reported by DelloStaffolo et al. (2004) for systems prepared with yogurts fortified with 1.3% w/v of different fiber sources (bamboo, inulin, apple, wheat).

The differences in rheological behavior of products derived from quince and from peach can be attributed to differences in chemical composition. The WSF of P and C products showed higher uronics and NCS content than MA and ME (Table 1). In addition, WSF and AIR of P presented the highest pectic polysaccharides estimation (Figure 2) and the WSF of P was highly polydisperse. It must be stated that Funami et al. (2007) reported that methyl cellulose aggregates in aqueous systems increased elastic modulus.

When comparing the ME with the MA system, both prepared with a 10% concentration, the greater consistency shown by the former could be explained by different reasons. From hydrodynamic view point, both fractions were polydisperse (Figure 5) but ME formed higher aggregates showing higher $Z_{average}$. Hwang and Kokini (1992) stated that flow parameters in pectin dilute solutions are directly related to the hydrodynamic volume of the molecule. On the other hand, in systems having a high concentration of particles, the resistance to deformation is no longer directly related to the concentration of the suspended particles, but to a controlling mechanism called "the crowding effect", which increases rapidly as concentration increases. Furthermore, the resistance to deformation becomes dependent on particle shape. Elongated particles will be much more prone to collide and form entanglements (Navarro et al., 1999). From chemical view point, ME showed more WSF and NCS content (Figure 1) than MA. In addition, WSF from ME was richer in uronics (Table 1), pectin and hemicellulosic polysaccharides than WSF from MA and ME presented higher DB (Figure 2B and Figure 3 E and F).

In order to evaluate the influence of chemical composition on rheological behavior, a correlation analysis was performed, taking into account the different concentrations of fractions P, C, MA, ME used for rheological characterization. The Pearson product moment correlation coefficients range from -1 (negative dependence) to +1 (positive dependence), and measure the strength of the linear relationship between the variables evaluated. Table 4 reports the most important results in the form of the coefficients for each pair of variables. It is also shown, in parentheses, the p value and the size of the sample. The exponent "n", from the power law equation describing G', was the only rheological parameter that was significantly correlated with the composition of the fractions. The AIR content, the hemicellulosic polysaccharide and the NCS content of WSF showed a significant and negative relationship with the parameter "n". Additionally, it was observed a significant and positive correlation for "n" and the inverse of WSF content and of pectin content of WSF. A non significant correlation was observed between n-exponent and DB (Table 4). From these analysis it could be concludedthat, in general, when more AIR, WSF and hemicellulosic polysaccharides, NCS and pectic polysaccharides were present in a water suspension, G' tended to become independent from frequency (ω) and therefore, less weak gel systems were obtained. According to Singthong et al. (2005), the increase in pectin concentration in fractions isolated from Krueo Ma Noy (*Cissampelospareira*) gives origin to higher gel strength for the hydrocolloid obtained.

Conclusion

Products enriched in DF and obtained from quince waste (MA, ME) and peach (P, C) were characterized.

The analysis of minerals present in the cell wall showed that Ca, K, P and Mg were the four most abundant elements. 5 g of DF can provide around 1.5-2% of the Ca dietary reference intake and 15-26% of the Fe dietary reference intake for males between 31 and 50 years, contributing to fiber nutritional value.

Fiber fractions obtained from peach showed a greater histological integrity than those obtained from quince, trend that can be ascribed to the fact that the former were obtained from less damaged tissues. This might help to the better performance of the peach fractions as DF.

Higher pectin content in P and C products and also in their respective water soluble fractions (WSF) were found. In addition, pectins from P and C were methylated and branched and WSF of P showed high polydispersity. MA and ME were less polydisperse but particles or aggregates of WSF of ME were greater.

Weak gels of similar mechanical spectra were obtained when 2% w/w suspensions of P or C or 10% w/w suspensions of fibers from quince waste were formulated. In general, when more alcohol insoluble residue, WSF, hemicellulosic polysaccharides, NCS or pectic polysaccharides were present in water suspensions, less weak gel systems were obtained. Carbohydrate characteristics, particle size distribution and polidispersity seemed to have a major influence on rheological behavior of water suspensions of products isolated.

It can be concluded that DF fractions obtained from quince waste and peach can be used as healthy ingredients that can act as rheology modifiers in food products.

Acknowledgments

The authors acknowledged the financial support from University of Buenos Aires (UBACyT EX-089, 20020100100726 and 20020130100550BA), University of IllesBalears (INIA, Ref: RTA2009-00118-C02), National Agency of Scientific and Technological Promotion of Argentina (ANPCyT-PICT 38239 and 2088) and National Scientific and

Technical Research Council of Argentina (CONICET-PIP 11220090100531 and 11220120100507CO01).

References

Alonso Mougán, M., Meijide, F., Jover, A., Rodrígues-Núñez, E.& Vázquez-Tato, J. (2002). Rheological behavior of an amide pectin. *Journal of Food Engineering*, *55*, 123-129.

AOAC International.(2006). Official Methods of Analysis of the Association of Official Analytical Chemists. USA: AOAC, Inc. *Method,941*, 12, Ash of Spices.

Arnous, A. & Meyer, A. (2009). Quantitative prediction of cell wall polysaccharide composition in grape (*Vitisvinífera* L.) and apple (*Malusdomestica*) skins from acid hydrolysis monosaccharide profiles. *Journal of Agriculture and Food Chemistry*, *57*, 3611-3619.

Augusto, P. E., Falguera, V., Cristianini, M.& Ibarz, A. (2011). Influence of fiber addition on the rheological properties of peach juice. *International Journal of Food Science and Technology*, *46*, 1086-1092.

Camino, N., Perez, O.& Pilosof, A. M. (2009). Molecular and functional modification of hydroxypropylmethylcellulose by high-intensity ultrasound. *Food Hydrocolloids*, *23*, 1089–1095.

Camino, N., Sánchez, C., Rodríguez Patino, J.&Pilosof, A. M. (2011). Hydroxypropylmethyl cellulose at the oil-water interface. Part I. Bulk behavior and dynamic adsorption as affected by pH. *Food Hydrocolloids*, *25*, 1-11.

de Escalada Pla, M., González, P., Sette, P., Portillo, F., Rojas, A. M. &Gerschenson, L. (2012). Effect of processing on physico-chemical characteristics of dietary fiber concentrates obtained from peach (PrunuspersicaL.) peel and pulp. *Food Research International*, *49*, 184-192.

de Escalada Pla, M. F., Ponce, N. M., Stortz, C. A., Gerschenson, L. N.& Rojas, A. M. (2007). Composition and functional properties of enriched fiber products obtained from pumpkin (*Cucurbitamoschata* Duchesne ex Poiret). LWT - *Food Science and Technology*, *40*, 1176-1185.

deEscaladaPla, M., Rojas, A. M.&Gerschenson, L. (2013). Effect of butternut (*Cucurbitamoschata* Duchesne ex Poiret) fibers on bread making, quality and staling. *Food and Bioprocess Technology*, *6*, 828-838.

de Escalada Pla, M., Uribe, M., Fissore, E., Gerschenson, L.& Rojas, A. M. (2010). Influence of the isolation procedure on the characteristics of fiber-rich products obtained from quince wastes. *Journal of Food Engineering*, *96*, 239-248.

Dello Staffolo, M., Bertola, N., Martino, M.& Bevilacqua, A. (2004). Influence of dietary fiber addition on sensory and rheological properties of yogurt. *International Dairy Journal*, *14*, 263-268.

Doublier, J. L.&Launay, B. (1981). Rheology of galactomannan solutions: comparative study of guar gum and locust bean gum. *Journal of Texture Studies*, *12*, 151–172.

Eim, V. S., Simal, S., Rosselló, C.&Femenia, A. (2008). Effects of addition of carrot dietary fiber on the ripening process of a dry fermented sausage (sobrassada). *Meat Science*, *80*, 173–182.

Elleuch, M., Bedigian, D., Roiseux, O., Besbes, S., Blecker, C.&Attia, H. (2011). Dietary fiber and fiber rich by-products of food processing: Characterisation, Technological functionality and commercial applications: A review. *Food Chemistry*, *124*, 411-421.

Elleuch, M., Besbes, S., Roiseux, O., Blecker, C., Deroanne, C., Drira, N.&Attia, H. (2008). Date flesh: Chemical composition and characteristics of the dietary fiber. *Food Chemistry*, *111*, 676-682.

Femenia, A., Lefebvre, A. C., Thebaudin, J. Y., Robertson, J.& Bourgeois, C. (1997). Physical and sensory properties of model foods supplemented with cauliflower fiber. *Journal of Food Science*, *62*, 1-7.

Femenia, A., Sánchez, E., Simal, S.&Rosselló, C. (1998a). Modification of cell wall composition of apricot (*Prunusarmeniaca*) during drying and storage under modified atmospheres. *Journal of Agriculture and Food Chemistry*, *46*, 5248-5253.

Femenia, A., Sánchez, E., Simal, S.&Rosselló, C. (1998b). Developmental and ripening-related effects on the cell wall of apricot (*Prunusarmeniaca*) fruit. *Journal of the Science of Food and Agriculture*, *77*, 487-493.

Filisetti-Cozzi, T. M. C. C.& Carpita, N. C. (1991). Measurement of uronic acids without interference from neutral sugars. *Analytical Biochemistry*, *197*, 157-162.

Fissore, E., Rojas, A. M.& Gerschenson, L. (2012). Rheological performance of pectin-enriched products isolated from red beet (*Beta vulgaris* L. var. *conditiva*) through alkaline and enzymatic treatments. *Food Hydrocolloids*, *26*, 249-260.

Food,& Nutrition Board, Institute of Medicine. (2001). Dietary reference intakes for Vitamin A, Vitamin K, arsenic, boron, chromium, copper, iodine, iron, manganese, molybdenum, nickel, silicon, vanadium and zinc. National Academy Press. Washington, DC.

Food and Nutrition Board, Institute of Medicine. (2005). Dietary reference intakes for water, potassium, sodium, chloride and sulfate. Washington, DC: National Academy Press.

Food and Nutrition Board, Institute of Medicine. (2011). Dietary reference intakes for calcium and Vitamin D. Washington, DC: National Academy Press.

Funami, T., Kataoka, Y., Hitoe, M., Asai, I., Takahashi, R. & Nishinari, K. (2007). Thermal aggregation of methylcellulose with different molecular weights. *Food Hydrocolloids*, *21*, 46–58.

Gómez, M., Ronda, F., Blanco, C., Caballero, P.&Apesteguía, A. (2003). Effect of dietary fiber on dough rheology and bread quality. *European Food Research and Technology*, *216*, 51–56.

González-Centeno, M. R., Rosselló, C., Simal, S., Garau, M. C., López, F.&Femenia, A.(2010). Physico-chemical properties of cell wall materials obtained from ten grape varieties and their byproducts: grape pomaces and stems. LWT - *Food Science and Technology*, *43*, 1580-1586.

Grigelmo-Miguel, N., Ibarz-Ribas, A.& Martin-Belloso, O. (1999). Rheology of peach dietary fiber suspensions. *Journal of Food Engineering*, *39*, 91-99.

Hwang, J.&Kokini, J. (1992). Contribution of the side branches to rheological properties of pectins. *Carbohydrate polymers*, *19*, 41-50.

Igartuburu, J., Pando, E., Rodriguez, L.& Gil-Serrano, A. (1997). An acidic xyloglucan from grape skins. *Phytochemistry*, *46*(8), 1307-1312.

Ikeda, S.&Nishinari, K. (2001). "Weak gel"-type rheological properties of aqueous dispersions of nonaggregated kappa-carrageenan helices. *Journal of Agricultural and Food Chemistry*, *49*, 4436-4441.

Jarvis, M. C. (2011). Plant cell walls: Supramolecular assemblies. *Food Hydrocolloids*, *25*, 257–262.

Kim, C.&Yoo, B. (2006). Rheological properties of rice starch-xanthan gum mixtures. *Journal of Food Engineering*, *75*, 120-128.

Manrique, G.&Lajolo, F. (2002). FT-IR spectroscopy as a tool for measuring degree of methyl esterification in pectins isolated from ripening papaya fruit. *Postharvest Biology and Technology*, *25*, 99-107.

McCann, M. C., Hammouri, M., Wilson, R., Belton, P.& Roberts, K. (1992). Fourier transform infrared microspectroscopy is new way to look at plant cell walls. *Plant Physiology*, *100*, 1940-1947.

Murphy, R. (1997). Static and dynamic light scattering of macromolecules: what can we learn? *Current Opinion in Biotechnology*, *8*, 25-30.

Navarro, A., Ferrero, C.&Zaritzky, N. (1999). Rheological characterization of "dulce de leche" by dynamic and steady shear measurements.*Journal of Texture Studies*, *30*, 43-58.

Ng, A.& Waldron, K. W. (1997).Effect of cooking and pre-cooking on cell wall chemistry in relation to firmness of carrot tissues. *Journal of the Science of Food and Agriculture*, *73*, 503-512.

Ngouémazong, D. E., Kabuye, G., Fraeye, I., Cardinaels, R., Van Loey, A., Moldenaers, P.&Hendrickx, M. (2012). Effect of debranching on the rheological properties of Ca^{2+}-pectin gels. *Food hydrocolloids*, *26*(1), 44-53.

Pornsak, S. (2003). Chemistry of Pectin and its Pharmaceutical Uses: A Review. *Silpakorn University International Journal*, *3*(1–2), 206-228.

Rodgers, J.&Nicewander, W. (1988). Thirteen ways to look at the correlation coefficient. *The American Statistician*, *42*, 59–66.

Saeman, J. F., Moore, W. E., Mitchell, R. L.& Millett, M. A. (1954).Techniques for the determination of pulp constituents by quantitative paper chromatography. *TAPPI*, *34*, 336-365.

Schieber, A., Stintzing, F. C.& Carle, R. (2001.)By-products of plant food processing as a source of functional compounds–recent developments. *Trends in Food Science and Technology*, *12*, 401–413.

Selvendran, R. R., March, J. F.& Ring, S. G. (1979). Determination of aldoses and uronic acid content of vegetable fiber. *Analytical Biochemistry*, *96*, 282-292.

Singthong, J., Ningsanond, S., Cui, S. W.& Goff, H. D. (2005). Extraction and physicochemical characterization of Krueo Ma Noy pectin. *Food Hydrocolloids*, *19*, 793-801.

Sokal, R.&Rohlf, F. J. (1980). Biometry. WH Freeman and Company, San Francisco, USA.

Soukoulis, C., Lebesi, D.&Tzia, C. (2009). Enrichment of ice cream with dietary fiber: Effects on rheological properties, ice crystallisation and glass transition phenomena. *Food Chemistry*, *115*, 665–671.

Van Buren, J. P. (1979). The chemistry of texture in fruits and vegetables. *Journal of Texture Studies*, *10*, 1-23.

In: Dietary Fiber
Editor: Marvin E. Clemens

ISBN: 978-1-63463-655-1
© 2015 Nova Science Publishers, Inc.

Chapter 7

CHARACTERIZATION OF FRACTIONS ENRICHED IN DIETARY FIBER OBTAINED FROM WASTE (LEAVES, STEMS, RHIZOMES AND PEELS) OF *BETA VULGARIS* INDUSTRIALIZATION

***Elizabeth Erhardt*[1], *Cinthia Santo Domingo*[1,2], *Ana Maria Rojas*[1,3], *Eliana Fissore*[1,3,4] *and Lía Gerschenson*[1,3,4] ***

[1]Department of Industry, School of Exact and Natural Sciences, Buenos Aires University, Argentina

[2]Fellow of the National Scientific and Technical Research Council (CONICET), Argentina

[3]Member of the National Scientific and Technical Research Council (CONICET), Argentina

[4]These authors contributed equally to the manuscript

ABSTRACT

According to many scientific studies, people who have a diet rich in fiber have a low incidence of gastrointestinal disorders, diabetes mellitus, obesity and cardiovascular disease. An alternative to compensate the deficiency of dietary fiber in foods is to incorporate it as a supplement.

Pectin is a fermentable dietary fiber as it resists digestion and absorption in the human small intestine and experiences a total or partial fermentation in the large intestine. Besides possessing multiple health benefits, pectin has applications in the food industry as a gelling agent, thickener, fat replacement, emulsion stabilizer, among others.

In the industry, pectin is usually extracted by treating the raw material (i.e., apple, citrus) with dilute mineral acid at pH near 2, generating large amounts of effluents in need of treatment. Enzymatic methods of pectin isolation are an environmentally friendly alternative to acidic methods usually used and allow labeling products with ecological

* Corresponding author. Departamento de Industrias, FCEN, UBA; Ciudad Universitaria, (1428) Buenos Aires. Argentina; Tel.: +541145763366; fax: +541145763366. E-mail address: lia@di.fcen.uba.ar (L. N. Gerschenson).

connotations tending to promote the consumption of products with these features. On the other hand, the increased consumption of fresh cut and peeled products generates a huge amount of wastes that is usually discarded; its use to obtain pectin can help to reduce pollution and restore biomass and nutrients.

The isolation techniques and characteristics of different fractions of dietary fiber isolated from industrialization wastes (leaves, stems, rhizomes and peels) of *Beta vulgaris* var. *conditiva* were studied in this research. The cell wall material was obtained through drying and grinding of *Beta vulgaris* wastes and its treatment with boiling ethanol rendered the alcohol insoluble residue. To isolate pectin enriched fractions, two different pre-treatments were assayed: one with sodium carbonate and another one with sodium hydroxide. The last one was selected because of the high yields and the product obtained was subjected to enzymatic digestion with cellulase and hemicellulase to obtain previously cited fractions. The highest antioxidant activity was detected in the cell wall material. The highest yield of the pectin enriched fractions was observed for the sodium hydroxide treatment followed by hydrolysis with cellulase. Rheological characterization showed pseudoplastic behavior with yield stress in flow assays. Dynamic assays showed weak gel behavior for all pectin enriched fractions in the presence of $CaCl_2$. Carbohydrate characteristics and polyphenol content influenced the antioxidant activity and rheological behavior.

Isolated fractions exhibited different technological characteristics and may be applied as food additives or ingredients.

INTRODUCTION

Dietary Fiber

According to the Codex Alimentarius (Miller Jones, 2014), dietary fiber is defined as "carbohydrate polymers with 10 or more monomeric units which are neither digested nor absorbed in the human small intestine including edible carbohydrate polymers naturally occurring in the food as consumed; edible carbohydrate polymers which have been obtained from food raw material by physical, enzymatic, or chemical means and which have a beneficial physiological effect demonstrated by generally accepted scientific evidence; edible synthetic carbohydrate polymers which have a beneficial physiological effect demonstrated by generally accepted scientific evidence".

The carbohydrate polymers of plant origin that meet the definition of fiber may be closely associated in the plant with lignin or other non-carbohydrate components such as phenolic compounds, waxes, saponins, phytates, cutin, phytosterols. These substances when closely associated with carbohydrate polymers of plant origin and extracted with them for analysis of fiber may be considered as part of them. However, when separated from the carbohydrate polymers and added to a food, these substances should not be considered as fiber (Miller Jones, 2014).

Based on their water solubility, dietary fiber may be divided into insoluble dietary fiber (IDF), which includes celluloses, some hemicelluloses and lignin and soluble dietary fiber (SDF), which includes β-glucans, pectins, gums, mucilages and some hemicelluloses. Approximately 75 % of fiber in food is, in general, present as insoluble fiber (Matos-Chamorro and Chambilla-Mamani, 2010). Some fruits, whole oat, barley, dried beans and other legumes are good sources of soluble fiber (Dreher, 1999, 2001).

The amount of fiber consumed varies geographically. In industrialized countries such as USA, fiber average consumption is 12 - 15 g/day, much lower than the World Health Organization fiber recommended intake of 25 - 40 g/day. On the other hand, some African communities are known to consume as much as 50 g of fiber daily (Jalili et al., 2007). According to Meisner et al. (2011), average dietary fiber consumption in Argentina is 15.3 g/day of which 10.26 g is insoluble fiber and 5.04 g soluble fiber.

Different investigations at laboratory level have concluded that dietary fiber has a protective role in diseases or conditions including appendicitis, hiatus hernia, diverticular disease, diabetes, colorectal cancer, hemorrhoids, inflammatory bowel diseases, renal calculi, gallstones, gastric and duodenal ulcers, virus diseases, atherosclerosis and ischemic heart disease (Chesson, 2006).

Antioxidants

An antioxidant may be defined as "any substance that when present at relatively low concentrations, compared to those of the oxidizable substrates, significantly delays or inhibits oxidation of that substrate" (Halliwell and Gutteridge, 1995). Increased intakes of dietary antioxidants may help to maintain an adequate antioxidant status, defined as the balance between antioxidants and oxidants in living organisms (Pulido et al., 2000).

Fruits and vegetables rich in pigments like carotenoids or betalains are important sources of antioxidants (Fernandez Lopez et al., 2010). Phenolic compounds have also shown antioxidant activity producing an inhibition of cancer cell proliferation, diminishing vascularization, protecting neurons against oxidative stress, stimulating the dilatation of blood vessels and promoting the insulin secretion due to their capacity to trap free radicals such as peroxide, hydroperoxide or lipid peroxyl present in biological systems (Pulido et al., 2000).

Dietary fiber present in edible plants shows approximately a 2.5 % content of associated polyphenols. The evaluation of the relation between dietary fiber and antioxidant activity can be useful to the more complete characterization of fiber and to evaluate its effect on health and its potential application as a food ingredient (Saura-Calixto, 2011; Palafox-Carlos et al., 2011).

Pectin

Some polysaccharides constituting dietary fiber have high water affinity and are referred to as soluble dietary fiber. Soluble dietary fiber includes pectic substances and a variety of gums and mucilages and comprises about 25 % of the dietary fiber consumed (Dreher, 1999).

Many health benefits attributed to dietary fiber appear to be a direct consequence of its ability to increase viscosity in the digestive tract. One of the most important physiological properties of soluble fibers is the ability to retain water which is attributed to the presence of sugar residues with free polar groups such as OH, COOH and C=O allowing hydrogen bond formation with adjacent water molecules.

Plant cells are characterized by the presence of a wall in which complex physicochemical and enzymatic processes occur. The primary cell wall is constituted by pectin, cellulose, hemicellulose and a small proportion of proteins and phenolic compounds. The more external layer of the cell wall is known as middle lamella and is essentially constituted by pectic material (Oechslin et al., 2003; Pérez et al., 2003). Pectins have an important role in the viscous resistance of the cell structure and they also control the porosity of the cell wall. Vincken et al. (2003) proposed that the cellulose-hemicellulose network of the cell wall is embedded in a pectin matrix.

Pectic substances are a polysaccharide family constituting the cell wall. They are highly versatile and their structure is not as well known as their functional properties. Homogalacturonan, rhamnogalacturonan-I (RG-I), and rhamnogalacturonan-II (RG-II) are the more common identified polysaccharides that constitute pectins. Yapo (2011) proposed a pectin structure model comprising at least 17 different monosaccharides, of which the galacturonic acid results to be the most abundant followed by galactose and arabinose. The content of pectin and the composition of pectic substances are different for the different plant tissues and also differ with the development stage of the plant (Lopes da Silva and Rao, 2006).

Pectins have a great capacity of water retention (Jalili et al., 2007) and can gel under adequate conditions. The consumption of soluble polysaccharides which increase the viscosity can delay and reduce the concentration of glucose in blood one hour after eating because of the restricted access of amylases to the substrate fact that delays the glucose liberation from starch producing that reduction. The addition of soluble polysaccharides in the diet reduces noticeably the levels of total cholesterol and LDL cholesterol in blood for normal people or people with hyper-cholesterolemia; this effect can be attributed to the fact that biliar acids instead of being reabsorbed in the ileum and returned to the liver are trapped by the soluble polysaccharides and excreted determining that the cholesterol is used for the synthesis of the missing biliar acids (Chesson, 2006).

Pectins as Food Additives

The main uses for pectins are as gelling agents, thickening agents and stabilizers in food (Lopes da Silva and Rao, 2006). High-methoxyl pectins form gels in acidic and high soluble solid conditions whereas in low-methoxyl pectins, gelation occurs in the presence of divalent ions such as calcium and, in general, with reduced soluble solid concentration being this capacity of great interest in low caloric value foods.

Pectin Extraction

Extraction conditions can alter pectin composition, structure and physiological properties. Pectin extraction from raw material is usually performed under acidic conditions (pH 1.5 - 3.0) and at high temperatures (70 – 90 ºC) using hydrochloric acid, nitric acid or sulfuric acid.

The pectin raw extract is then separated from the residue by filtration or centrifugation and pectin is separated from the extract by precipitation with alcohol or by precipitation with an insoluble salt by addition of a polyvalent cation, usually aluminum. The precipitate obtained is washed with alcohol and pressed to remove soluble impurities, and finally dried and milled to yield powdered pectin (Lopes da Silva and Rao, 2006).

The use of non-pectolytic enzymes for pectin extraction is an alternative to industrial acidic extraction but, according to Endress et al. (2005), the combined use of cellulases and hemicellulases does not allow to obtain pectin yields as high as those achieved with traditional extraction. These enzymatic techniques have been described in bibliography but they have been rarely applied at industrial level due to the high costs involved. However, the acidic conditions used by the industry generate a high amount of effluents and their treatment represents an additional cost that revalorizes enzymatic procedures as environmentally friendly alternatives that allow obtaining green labeled products. It must be also considered that the different techniques might also produce pectins with different physicochemical and functional properties.

Industrial Residues

The food industry produces large volumes of wastes, both solids and liquids, resulting from the production, preparation, and consumption of food. These wastes pose increasing disposal and potentially severe pollution problems and represent a loss of valuable biomass and nutrients. Sub-products of vegetable processing represent an important issue for food industry (Laufenberg et al., 2003). Many researchers are studying the conversion of these residues into value added products (Makris et al., 2007). Some examples include the obtaining of pectins from sugar beet pomace, sunflower head residues, and olive pomace (Lopes da Silva and Rao, 2006).

Annual pectin consumption is estimated in 45×10^6 kg (Willats et al., 2006). Transformation of vegetable residues into value added products such as pectin would contribute to reduce pollution and to recover nutrients and biomass (Laufenberg et al., 2003).

The objectives of the present work are:

- to reduce the amount of residues from the processing of *Beta vulgaris* L. var *conditiva* (leaves, stems, rhizomes and peels) through their use for isolation of dietary fiber,
- to develop a method for pectin extraction which is less pollutant than the traditional industrial methods,
- to characterize the fractions obtained in order to determine their possible applications as food additives or ingredients.

Materials and Methods

Beta vulgaris L. var. *conditiva* Processing. Cell Wall Material

Beta vulgaris L. var. *conditiva* bought in a local market was washed and peeled. The edible root was separated and the leaves, stems, peels and rhizomes were dried in a convection oven (80 °C, 2.5 h, air rate: 0.5 m/s), milled in a domestic grinder (Connoísserve, China) and sieved (420 – 740 μm) to obtain the cell wall material (CWM) powder which was stored at -18 °C under vacuum into heat sealed Cryovac (polyvinyl chloride-polyvinylidene chloride copolymer) bags until usage.

Preparation of Alcohol - Insoluble Residue (AIR)

According to Martín-Cabrejas et al. (1994), 100 g of CWM were suspended in 350 ml of 80 % (v/v) ethanol solution and then boiled for 30 min under stirring. The residue obtained was then extracted with other 350 ml of 80 % (v/v) ethanol solution under boiling, for 15 min and twice with 250 ml of 80 % (v/v) ethanol boiling solution for 15 min. The insoluble residue was separated and washed with 100 ml of 80 % (v/v) ethanol and finally with 96 % (v/v) ethanol. Between each ethanol treatment, the suspension was filtered and the solvent was discarded. The material was left overnight under lab hood to eliminate the ethanol and the ethanol free product was freeze-dried (Stokes freeze-drier, Stokes Company, Philadelphia, MA, USA) after freezing with liquid nitrogen. The product was then milled (Wemir E909, Argentina) and stored at -18 °C under vacuum into heat sealed Cryovac (polyvinyl chloride-polyvinylidene chloride copolymer) bags until usage.

Isolation of Pectin Enriched Fractions

Considering that beetroot tissue contains ferulic acid which cross-links pectin macromolecules through arabinose residues to anchor them into the cell wall network, two pre-treatments prior to enzymatic digestion were evaluated in order to break ferulic acid bonds for obtaining adequate yields of polysaccharides:

- Carbonate pre-treatment (CO): 2.5 g AIR in 125 ml of 50 mM Na_2CO_3 solution were incubated for 30 min at room temperature with constant agitation. The product was filtered using glass fiber.
- Hydroxide pre-treatment (B): 2.5 g AIR in 125 ml of 2M NaOH solution were incubated for 30 min at room temperature with constant agitation. The product was filtered using glass fiber.

Also non pre-treated (NT) samples were evaluated.

Products obtained after pre-treatments or without pre-treatment, were subjected to the following enzymatic digestions:

- Hemicellulase (H): 10 g AIR with 0.25 g of hemicellulase H2125 (Sigma, St. Louis, USA) from Aspergillus niger in 1000 ml of 50mM sodium citrate buffer (pH 5.2).
- Cellulase (C): 10 g AIR with 0.05 g of cellulase C9422 (Sigma, St. Louis, USA) of Trichoderma viride in 1000 ml of 50mM sodium citrate buffer (pH 5.2).
- No enzymatic treatment (NE): 10 g AIR in 1000 ml of 50mM sodium citrate buffer (pH 5.2).

Hydrolysis was performed with constant stirring (10 rad s^{-1}) for 5 hours at 40 °C. Each system was filtered through glass fiber filter and two volumes of ethanol 96 % (v/v) were added to the supernatant to precipitate the soluble fiber. After filtration through glass fiber filter, the solid residue was freeze-dried under the conditions previously described.

Pectin enriched fractions obtained were named as follows:

- CO-NE: with carbonate pre-treatment and with no enzymatic treatment.
- CO-H: with carbonate pre-treatment and with hemicellulase.
- CO-C: with carbonate pre-treatment and with cellulase.
- B-NE: with hydroxide pre-treatment and with no enzymatic treatment.
- B-H: with hydroxide pre-treatment and with hemicellulase.
- B-C: with hydroxide pre-treatment and with cellulase.
- NT-NE: without pre-treatment and with no enzymatic treatment.
- NT-H: without pre-treatment and with hemicellulase.
- NT-C: without pre-treatment and with cellulase.

Chemical Analyses

Determination of Cellulose, Lignin and Non-Cellulose Carbohydrates in CWM and AIR

Hydrolysis of cellulose and non-cellulosic polysaccharides was performed according to Ng et al. (1998) by dispersion of ≈ 0.3000 g of sample product into 2080 μl of 72 %-sulfuric acid solution (v/v) for 3 h at room temperature. This dispersion was made 1 M-sulfuric acid by addition of enough deionized water (until 25.00 ml-final volume) and each sample was heated at 100 °C for 2.5 h in a water-bath. After this, all dispersions were cooled, centrifuged at 12,000g for 10 min and the supernatant was separated, carefully neutralized and total carbohydrate content was determined by the phenol–sulfuric method (Dubois et al., 1956). The residue was washed three times with deionized water, centrifuged at 12,000g for 10 min and, finally, freeze-dried. The residue obtained was weighed and reported as lignin.

A second procedure was carried out with other portion of ≈ 0.3000 g of each sample dispersed into 2080 μl of 72 %-sulfuric acid solution and water was immediately added up to 1 M-concentration followed by 2.5 h of heating at 100 °C. The final residue corresponded to cellulose + lignin.

The third hydrolysis-procedure was performed with a new portion of each sample following the technique applied for the second procedure, but 1 h of heating at 100 °C in a water-bath was applied in this case. Only the supernatant was separated for quantification as it was above indicated and uronic acid content was determined spectrophotometrically by the method reported by Filisetti-Cozzi and Carpita (1991).

Total Carbohydrates

The total carbohydrate content was evaluated according to the colorimetric method of Dubois et al. (1956) using phenol - sulfuric acid and measuring the absorbance at 490 nm. Galacturonic acid was used as standard.

Uronic Acids

Uronic acid content was determined through the spectrophotometric method reported by Filisetti-Cozzi and Carpita (1991), adding sulfamic acid - potassium sulfamate to the samples before heating with a sulfuric acid-tetraborate mixture, to suppress the browning of monosaccharides that were liberated.

Starch

Starch content was determined according to AACC (2000), using α-amylase and amyloglucosidase (Sigma starch kit, St. Louis, USA).

Neutral Sugars

Neutral sugars were calculated as the difference between total carbohydrate content and the sum of galacturonic acid and starch.

Proteins

The protein content in samples was determined according to Lowry et al. (1951) using bovine serum albumin (BSA) as standard.

Total Polyphenols

Total polyphenols were assayed using Folin-Ciocalteau reagent (Singleton and Rossi, 1965). Results are expressed as gallic acid equivalents (GAE) in g/100g.

Methanol

Methanol content was determined by the spectrophotometric method of Wood and Siddiqui (1971). Degree of methylation (DM) was calculated as the percent ratio between moles of methanol and moles of galacturonic acid in the analyzed sample.

Acetyl Groups

Acetyl groups were determined according to the method of Naumenko and Phillipov (1992).

Degree of acetylation (DA) was calculated as the percent ratio between moles of acetyl group and moles of galacturonic acid in the samples.

Antioxidant Activity

DPPH (diphenyl-2-picrylhydrazyl) assay was performed on CWM and AIR according to Brand-Williams et al. (1994). The antioxidant activity determined through the DPPH assay allows determining the ability of sample compounds to act as free radical scavengers or hydrogen donors. Ascorbic acid was used as standard and results were expressed as g sample / g DPPH. The anti-radical activity is defined as the amount of antioxidant necessary to decrease the initial DPPH concentration by 50 % (Efficient Concentration, EC_{50}). The anti-radical power (ARP) is defined as 1 / EC_{50} and the larger the ARP, the more efficient the antioxidant.

The ferric reducing antioxidant power (FRAP) assay was carried out according to the procedure described by Benzie and Strain (1996). This method measures the antioxidant capacity to reduce the Fe^{3+}/tripyridyl-s-triazine (TPTZ) complex, to the ferrous form. A $FeSO_4$ standard curve was prepared and results were expressed as μmol $FeSO_4$ / g sample.

Rheological Characterization

Systems containing a 2.00 % (w/v) concentration of the pectin enriched fractions were used for comparison of their rheological behavior. Around 0.0400 g of each material was suspended in 1700 μl of deionized water and vortexed until complete hydration. Solutions were heated in a water bath at 65 °C until dissolution. Total volume was completed to 2000 μl with $CaCl_2$ aqueous solution at 65 °C (40 mg Ca^{2+}/g pectin) while vortexing. Then, systems were stored at 25 °C for 18 hours to attain swelling equilibrium before measurement.

Rheological characterization was performed at 25 °C using a MCR300 Paar Physica (shear) rheometer (Anton Paar, Austria) equipped with a serrated parallel plate (PP35, Haake, Karlsruhe, Germany) geometry (35 mm-diameter). Temperature was maintained constant with a Peltier system. A gap size of 500 μm was set. Data points were recorded at steady-state.

Flow Assays

The flow behavior was determined at 25 °C in the 0.001 - 100 s^{-1} shear rate ($\dot{\gamma}$) range.

Ostwald's law (1) and Herschel-Bulkley model (2) were considered in the present work:

$$\tau = k\dot{\gamma}^n \quad (1)$$

wherein τ represents the shear stress, k represents the consistency index, and n is the flow index.

$$\tau = \tau_0 + k\dot{\gamma}^n \quad (2)$$

wherein τ represents the shear stress, τ_0 represents the yield stress, k represents the consistency index, and n is the flow index.

Dynamic Assays

Amplitude (stress versus strain) sweeps were first performed at constant frequency (0.1 Hz) and at constant temperature (25 °C) in order to determine the linear viscoelastic range (LVR) for each system, from which the value of strain to subsequently record the mechanical spectra (frequency sweeps) was selected. Each mechanical spectrum was then recorded at this constant strain value in the LVR: storage modulus (G') and loss modulus (G"), as well as the tangent of the phase angle (tan δ = G"/G') were obtained as a function of increasing angular frequency (ω) from 0 to 1000 rad s^{-1}, after reaching steady state condition for each point.

Statistical Analyses

Non-linear fittings and statistical evaluation were performed through Prism 5 Statistical Software for Windows (GraphPad, USA).

RESULTS AND DISCUSSION

Fractions Enriched in Dietary Fiber Form *Beta Vulgaris* L. var. *Conditiva* Residues

Yield

The yield of CWM was 8.80 g of powder / 100 g beetroot residues and the yield of AIR obtained from the CWM was 59.35 g /100 g CWM (dry basis). Fissore et al. (2007) reported a yield of 3.0 g CWM /100 g of pumpkin (*Cucurbita moschata*) mesocarp and in an additional paper published in 2011, the authors reported a yield of 2.4 g CWM /100 g beetroot mesocarp with a yield of 69.7 g AIR /100 g.

Chemical Characterization

Both CWM and AIR were mainly composed by carbohydrates (Table 1). For CWM, 57 % of total carbohydrates were constituted by cellulose and 15 % by uronic acids. For AIR, 44 % of total carbohydrates were cellulose and 20 % were uronic acids. The degree of methylation was 65 % for CWM and 42 % for AIR. The degree of acetylation was 71 % for CWM and 27 % for AIR. Lignin contents of 6.50 and 7.65 g / 100 g were observed in CWM and AIR, respectively. Proteins represented 19.3 g / 100 g CWM and 23 g / 100 g AIR.

Table 1. Chemical composition of CWM and AIR from *Beta vulgaris* L. var. *conditiva* residues

Composition	CWM	AIR
Total carbohydrates (g/100g)	71.4 ± 6.3[1]	98.2 ± 7.6[2]
Uronic acids (g/100g)	10.4 ± 0.7[1]	19.5 ± 3.9[2]
Cellulose (g/100g)	40.44 ± 0.06[1]	43.5 ± 1.1[2]
Other carbohydrates (g/100g)	20.56[1,3]	35.20[2,3]
Lignin (g/100g)	6.5 ± 0.3[1]	7.65 ± 0.07[2]
Proteins (g/100g)	19.3 ± 1.8[1]	23 ± 3[2]
Total polyphenols (g/100g)	1.1 ± 0.1[1]	0.80 ± 0.02[2]
Methanol (g/100g)	1.23 ± 0.02[1]	1.48 ± 0.05[2]
Degree of Methylation (%)	65	42
Acetyl groups (g/100g)	1.81 ± 0.04[1]	1.31 ± 0.03[2]
Degree of Acetylation (%)	71	27

[1]: expressed as g/100g CWM.
[2]: expressed as g/100g AIR.
[3]: calculated by difference.
DM and DA were calculated as the percent ratio between moles of methanol or acetyl group and moles of uronic acids, respectively.
CWM: cell wall material, AIR: alcohol insoluble residue.

Fissore et al. (2011) studied the chemical composition of the AIR of beetroot mesocarp (edible root) and reported a total carbohydrate content of 107 g / 100 g AIR, an uronic content of 13.7 g / 100 g AIR, a lignin content of 6.5 g / 100 g AIR, a cellulose content of 55 g / 100 g AIR and a protein content of 7.1 g / 100 g AIR.

Total polyphenol concentration (Table 1) found in CWM and AIR was 1.1 g / 100 g and 0.80 g / 100 g, respectively, being these values in the same order of those reported by Latorre et al. (2013) for beetroot mesocarp AIR.

Antioxidant Activity

Both CWM and AIR had a slow reaction with DPPH, reaching the stationary state in between 75 - 220 min for CWM and 180 - 410 min for AIR for the substrate concentration used. Reaction kinetic was faster for CWM than for AIR (Figure 1).

In Figure 2 it can be observed the EC_{50} value for CWM (EC_{50} = 87 g / g DPPH) and AIR (EC_{50} = 319 g / g DPPH). Jiménez-Escrig et al. (2003) studied the antioxidant activity of aqueous artichoke fractions and reported an EC_{50} value higher than the one observed in the present work for CWM but lower than the value obtained for AIR.

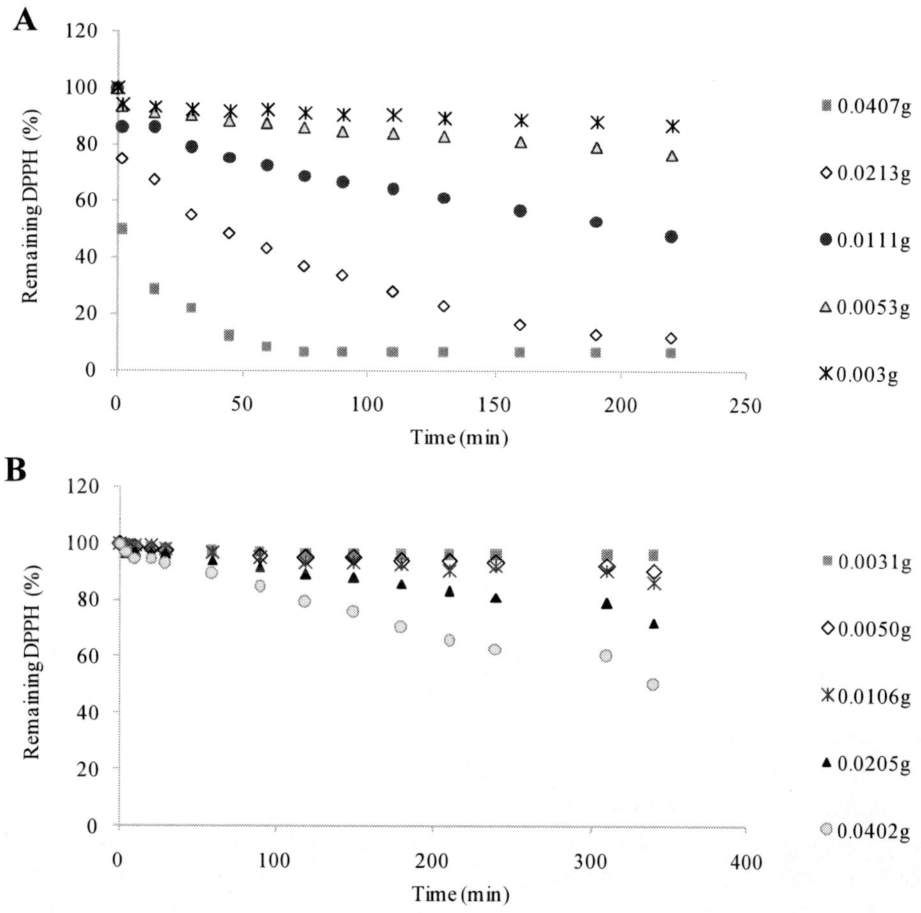

Figure 1. Kinetics of DPPH decay for (A) CWM and (B) AIR obtained from *Beta vulgaris* L. var. *conditiva* residues.

The CWM showed a higher antioxidant activity than AIR. The anti-radical power for CWM was 0.01 g DPPH / g sample and for AIR 0.003 g DPPH / g sample. Brand-Williams et al. (1994) reported an anti-radical power of 0.002 g DPPH / g sample for phenol, 2.33 g DPPH / g sample for ferulic acid and 12.5 g DPPH / g sample for gallic acid. Results obtained in the present work indicated that both CWM and AIR had a higher anti-radical power than phenol but lower than gallic and ferulic acids.

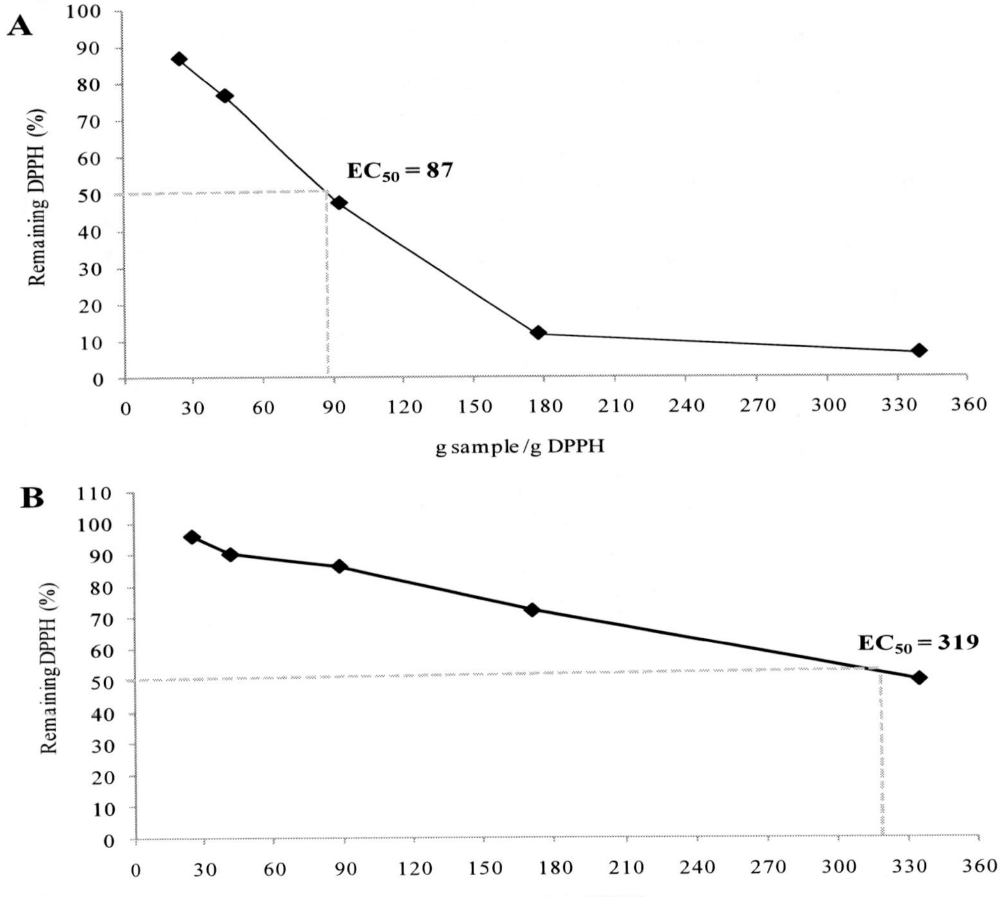

Figure 2. Relationship between remaining DPPH (%) and g sample / g DPPH for (A) CWM and (B) AIR from *Beta vulgaris* L. var. *conditiva* residues.

As it can be observed in Table 2, for FRAP assay, the CWM showed higher antioxidant activity (16.8 μmol Fe(II)/ g) than the AIR (9,6 μmol Fe(II) / g). Fuentes et al. (2013) studied the antioxidant properties of the peel and pulp of green and mature tomatoes. The results obtained for the pulp were 22 μmol Fe(II) / g and 32 μmol Fe(II) / g for green and mature tomatoes, respectively, and for the peel, the values obtained were 24 μmol Fe(II) / g and 47 μmol Fe(II) / g for green and mature tomatoes, respectively. Lianda et al. (2012) studied the antioxidant properties of honeys and the results obtained were between 34.99 and 408.14 mol Fe(II) / 100 g.

Table 2. Antioxidant activity determined through FRAP assay for cell wall material (CWM) and alcohol insoluble residue (AIR) of *Beta vulgaris* L. var. *conditiva* residues. Values determined after 90 min and expressed as mean values ± SD (n=2)

	Antioxidant capacity (μmol Fe (II) / g)
CWM	16.8 ± 1.2
AIR	9.60 ± 0.95

In Figure 3 it can be observed that the FRAP reaction kinetics were similar for both CWM and AIR.

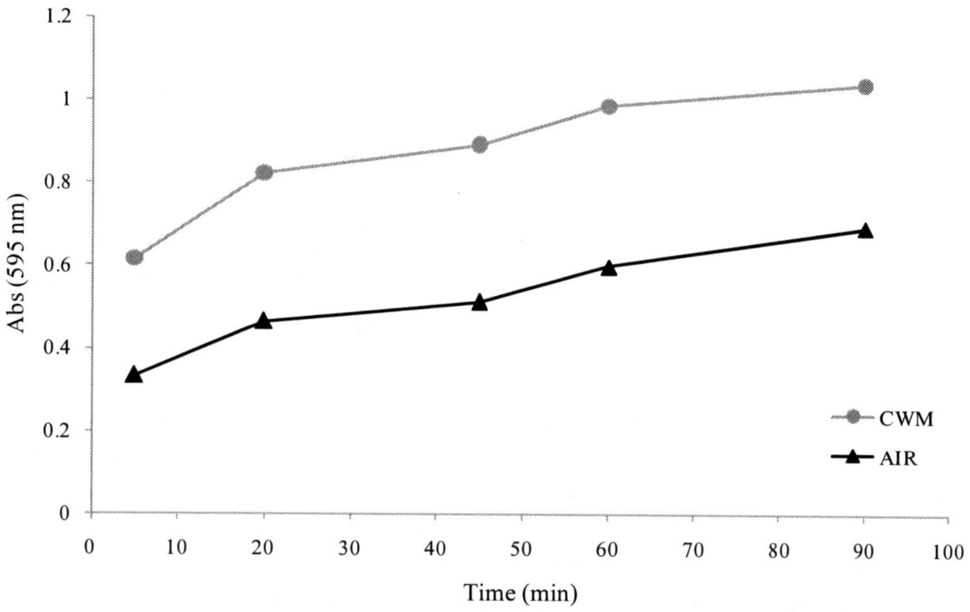

Figure 3. FRAP reaction kinetics for CWM and AIR of *Beta vulgaris* L. var. *conditiva* residues.

Pectin Enriched Fractions Obtained from the AIR of *Beta Vulgaris* L. Var. *Conditiva* Residues

Yield

Yields of fractions enriched in pectin were between 0.78 and 1.14 g/100g AIR for those isolated without a pre-treatment, less than 1 g/100g AIR for fractions isolated with a carbonate pre-treatment and between 26.17 and 44.83 g/100g AIR for fractions isolated with a hydroxide pre-treatment (Table 3).

Table 3. Yields of pectin enriched fractions isolated from AIR of *Beta vulgaris* residues without a pre-treatment (NT), through a carbonate pre-treatment (CO) and through hydroxide pre-treatment (B) followed by enzymatic digestion with hemicellulase (H), cellulase (C) or without enzyme (NE)

Fraction	Yield (g/100g AIR)
NT-NE	0.82
NT-H	1.14
NT-C	0.78
CO-NE	0.33
CO-H	0.42
CO-C	0.04
B-NE	26.17
B-H	29.85
B-C	44.83

Low yields for fractions isolated without a pre-treatment showed that enzymatic digestions were not adequate for an efficient extraction of pectin enriched fractions from beetroot stems, leaves, rhizomes and peels. Waldron et al. (1997) reported the presence of diferulate in beetroot pectic polysaccharides. As a consequence, low yields obtained for fractions isolated without a pre-treatment or with a carbonate pre-treatment could be attributed to the crosslinking of pectins by ferulic acid through ester bonds in terminal residues of their side chains (Fry, 1986) which might prevent polysaccharide separation. Dimerization can occur forming diferulates and contributing to the crosslinking of pectic polymers. On the other hand, hydroxide pre-treatment was effective in the saponification of diferulic bonds, allowing the isolation of pectin enriched fractions with yields between 26 and 45 g / 100 g AIR (Table 3).

Fissore et al. (2009) isolated pectin enriched fractions from pumpkin mesocarp through a digestion (30 °C, 20 h) with 0.25 g hemicellulase / 10 g CWM and 0.05 g cellulase / 10 g CWM and obtained yields of 4.7 and 6.12 g / 100 g CWM respectively; they also isolated pectin fractions from beetroot mesocarp using a basic pre-treatment which was followed by digestion with 0.75 g hemicellulase / 10 g CWM and 0.15 g cellulase / 10 g CWM and the yields obtained were 8.2 g / 100 g CWM for hemicellulase treatment and 15.2 g / 100 g CWM for cellulase treatment, being these values comparable to those obtained in the present work from AIR. Nawirska and Kwasniewska (2005) isolated pectin enriched fractions from apple pomace, pears and carrots with yields of 11.7, 13.4 and 3.88 g / 100 g CWM, respectively. Selvendran (1985) isolated pectin enriched fractions from apples and sugar beets through different extraction methods obtaining yields between 10 and 20.9 g / 100 apple CWM and 7.4 and 23 g / 100 g sugar beet CWM, depending on the extraction method applied.

Due to the low yields obtained in the present work for fractions isolated through NT and CO pre-treatments, it was decided to continue the following studies only with fractions isolated through pre-treatment B.

Chemical Composition

As it can be observed in Table 4, pectin enriched fractions were mainly constituted by carbohydrates (57.95 – 72.49 g / 100 g). Uronic acids concentrations were between 39.16 and 59.78 g / 100 g. Starch content differed between the three fractions being less than 1 g / 100 g for fraction B-C and 17.5 g / 100 g for fraction B-H. Fissore (2009) determined higher starch content in pectin enriched fractions isolated through hemicellulase (H2125, Sigma) digestion of pumpkin and beetroot mesocarp and suggested that hemicellulose degradation would allow the liberation of starch physically retained in the cellulose - xyloglucan network or other hemicelluloses in the cell wall. Neutral sugars concentration took values between 10.35 and 18.35 g / 100 g. Proteins were important components in both CWM and AIR (Table 3), whereas in pectin enriched fractions protein concentration was approximately 3 g / 100 g (Table 4). All fractions had low degree of methylation (< 50 %) and acetylation and these low values could be ascribed to the hydroxide pre-treatment performed.

Total polyphenols took values between 0.21 and 0.24 g / 100 g. These values were lower than those observed for CWM and AIR, which could be ascribed to the hydroxide pre-treatment performed (Martinez et al., 2012). Since polyphenols are the main source of antioxidant activity, and considering the low polyphenol content in fractions, it was decided not to evaluate their antioxidant activity.

Fraction B-H contained a higher starch content which limits its industrial application in the development of products where it is necessary a low glycemic value.

Table 4. Chemical composition of *Beta vulgaris* pectin enriched fractions isolated through a hydroxide (B) pre-treatment followed by hydrolysis with hemicellulase (H), cellulase (C) or without enzyme (NE)

Composition	B-NE	B-H	B-C
Total Carbohydrates (g/100g)	72.49 ± 3.99	70.57 ± 1.24	57.95 ± 3.29
Uronic Acids (g/100g)	56.53 ± 3.00	59.78 ± 3.10	39.16 ± 1.77
Starch (g/100g)	5.61 ± 0.01	17.54 ± 0.18	0.441 ± 0.042
Neutral Sugars (g/100g)	10.35	13.25	18.35
Proteins (g/100g)	3.54 ± 0.24	3.26 ± 0.03	3.35 ± 0.10
Total Polyphenols (g/100g)	0.24 ± 0.03	0.21 ± 0.01	0.208 ± 0.003
Methanol (g/100g)	0.033± 0.004	0.008± 0.004	0.005± 0.002
DM (%)[1]	0.32	0.11	0.07
Acetyl Groups (g/100g)	1.91 ± 0.22	2.64 ± 0.21	3.02 ± 0.02
DA (%)[2]	0.264 ± 0.03	0.256 ± 0.020	0.289 ± 0.019

DM: Degree of Methylation, DA: Degree of Acetylation.

DM[1] and DA[2] were calculated as a percent ratio between moles of methanol or acetyl group and moles of uronic acids, respectively.

Yapo (2009) characterized pectin enriched fractions isolated from yellow passion fruit rind through three different methods: alcohol precipitation, dialysis and metal-ion precipitation. The authors observed lower yields than those obtained in the present work, with the highest yield (7.5 g / 100 g) for fraction isolated through alcohol precipitation.

Rheological Properties

Flow Behavior

As can be observed in Figure 4, for calcium systems, viscosity decreased with shear rate increase showing a typical pseudoplastic behavior. Herschel-Bulkley models were used to fit data because all systems showed yield stress (τ_0). System B-C showed the highest flow index (n) indicating a less pseudoplastic behavior for this fraction when compared to fractions B-NE and B-H. System B-C also showed the highest yield stress value and consistency index (k) (Table 5).

Table 5. Herschel Bulkley parameters for calcium systems

	n	τ_0 (Pa)	k (Pa s^n)	R^2
B-NE	0.49	78.05	55.09	0.97
B-H	0.49	94.33	44.29	0.94
B-C	0.63	126.2	30.72	0.92

n: flow index, τ_0: yield stress, k: consistency index, R^2: goodness of fitting (α: 0.05).
Fraction B-NE: hydroxide pre-treatment and no enzymatic treatment.
Fraction B-H: hydroxide pre-treatment and hemicellulase treatment.
Fraction B-C: hydroxide pre-treatment and cellulase treatment.

Viscoelastic Behavior

Systems containing calcium were studied through dynamic rheology. Amplitude sweeps were performed to determine the linear viscoelastic region, where there is a linear dependence between strain and shear stress. A strain of 1.00 % was selected to perform dynamic assays.

Mechanical spectra for all systems (Figure 5) showed G' > G" in one order of magnitude which is characteristic of true biopolymer gels (Doublier et al., 1992). It was also observed a slight frequency dependence for G' and G" which indicates weak gel behavior for all systems. The low degree of methylation of isolated pectin enriched fractions determined their gelling capacity in the presence of calcium. It can be observed a cross-over tendency for G' and G" at high frequencies. Gels obtained are physical gels in which hydrated pectin macromolecules relate to each other through hydrogen bonds and also through calcium coordination bonds. According to Vu et al. (2010), the yield stress determined through flow assays in pectin fractions is an expression of the solid behavior which can be confirmed through dynamic assays.

Sample isolated through cellulase hydrolysis showed lower values of G' and G" than the other samples. It also showed the cross-over between G' and G" at lower frequencies (Figure 5). This indicates that sample B-C constituted the weakest gel. This fraction had the lowest total carbohydrate and the highest neutral sugar contents. Neutral sugars are the expression of branches in pectin molecule and they could hinder gel formation in the presence of calcium (Ngouémazong et al., 2012).

According to rheological results obtained it can be concluded that fractions isolated through a hydroxide pre-treatment are potentially useful as additives for dairy and confectionary industries.

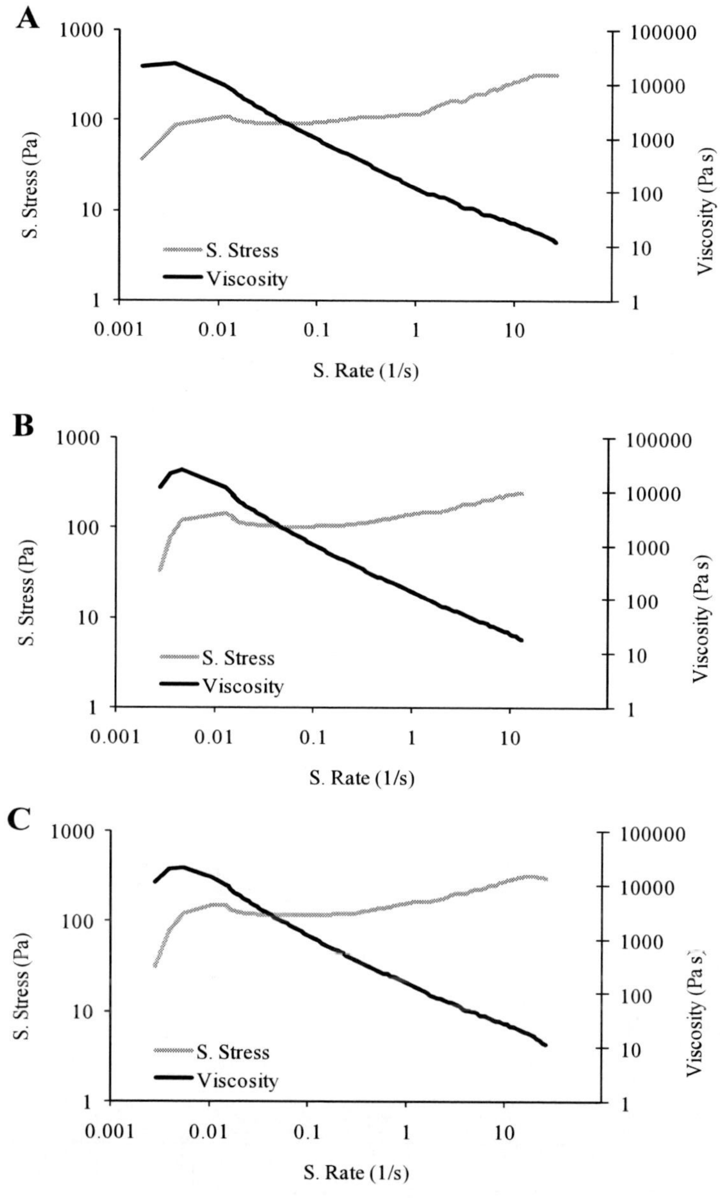

Figure 4. Flow behavior (25 °C) of aqueous systems containing pectin enriched fractions (2.00 % w/w) in the presence of calcium.
(A) Fraction B-NE: hydroxide pre-treatment and no enzymatic treatment
(B) Fraction B-H: hydroxide pre-treatment and hemicellulase treatment
(C) Fraction B-C: hydroxide pre-treatment and cellulase treatment.

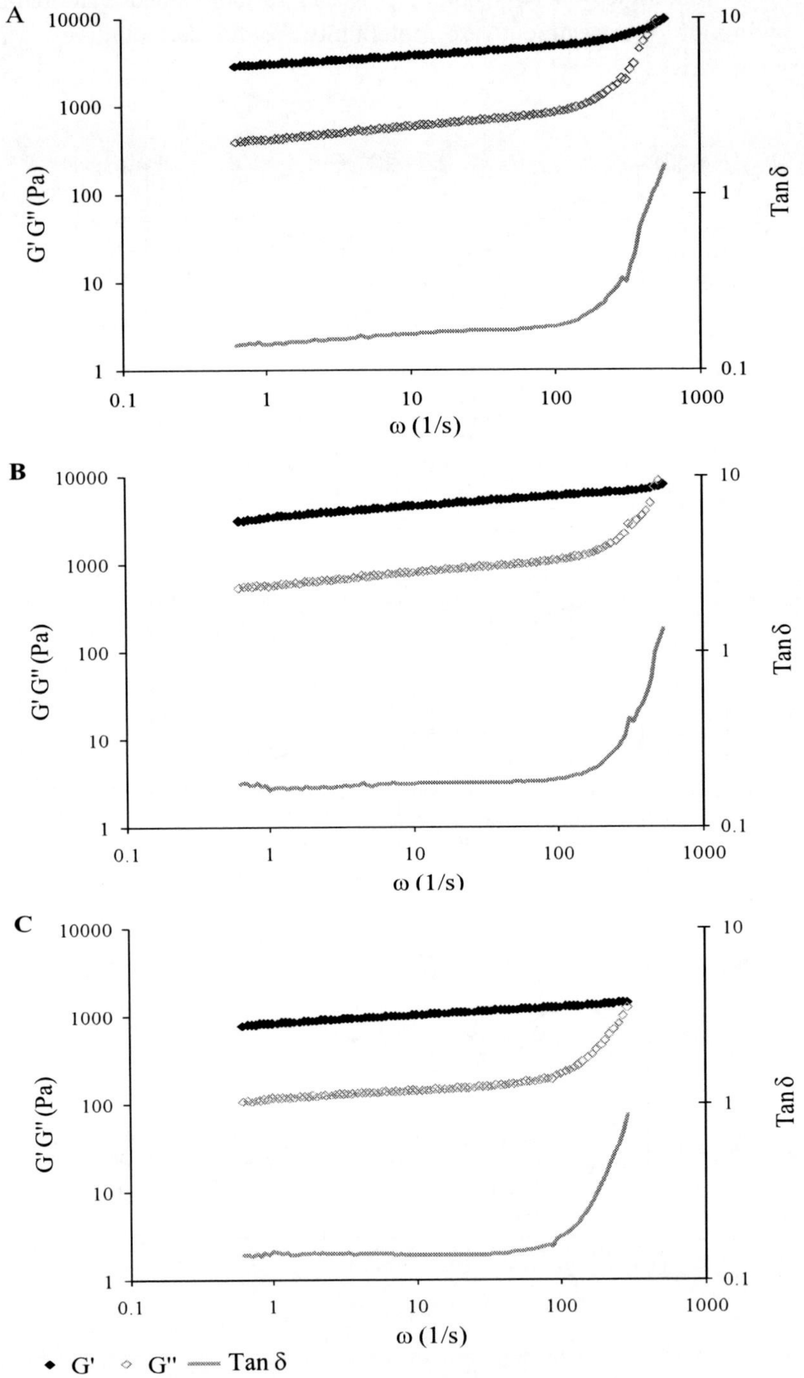

Figure 5. Mechanical spectra (25°C) of gels constituted by aqueous systems containing pectin enriched fractions (2.00 % w/w) in the presence of calcium.

Fraction B-NE: hydroxide pre-treatment and no enzymatic treatment.

Fraction B-H: hydroxide pre-treatment and hemicellulase treatment.

Fraction B-C: hydroxide pre-treatment and cellulase treatment.

CONCLUSION

Simple techniques involving procedures of dehydration, milling and/or ethanol treatment allowed the isolation of dietary fiber enriched fractions (CWM, AIR) from residues of *Beta vulgaris* L. var. *conditiva* industrialization; these fractions showed a high content of carbohydrates and polyphenols and antioxidant activity.

The hydroxide pre-treatment of the alcohol insoluble residue, followed by acidic treatment at pH 5.2 or acidic and enzymatic (cellulase, hemicellulase) treatment, allowed obtaining pectin enriched fractions with diverse properties. Pectin fraction isolated through hydroxide pre-treatment and hemicellulase digestion (yield ≈ 30 %), presented the highest starch content which could limit its use in the development of healthy food. Pectin fraction isolated through hydroxide pre-treatment and no enzymatic digestion (yield ≈ 26 %) presented an important uronic acid content. The highest yield (45 %) was obtained applying the hydroxide pre-treatment followed by cellulase digestion.

Pseudoplastic flow behavior with yield stress was observed for all pectin aqueous systems in the presence of calcium. Dynamic assays for these systems revealed a weak gel behavior. The weakest gel behavior corresponded to the fraction isolated through hydroxide pre-treatment and cellulase digestion probably due to the lowest carbohydrate and the highest neutral sugar contents.

It can be concluded that methods developed for the use of residues of *Beta vulgaris* industrialization gave origin to fractions that could have different applications in the food industry. CWM and AIR can be used as functional ingredients for dietary fiber and antioxidant supplementation and pectin enriched fractions can be used as thickening and gelling agents in the presence of calcium. The obtaining of these useful fractions adds value to the raw material under study and contributes to the diminishing of environment pollution.

ACKNOWLEDGMENTS

The authors acknowledged the financial support from University of Buenos Aires (20020100100726 and 20020130100550BA), National Agency of Scientific and Technological Promotion of Argentina (ANPCyT-PICT 38239 and 2088) and National Scientific and Technical Research Council of Argentina (CONICET-PIP 11220090100531 and 11220120100507CO01).

REFERENCES

A.A.C.C. (2000). Approved methods of the AACC. Method 76.13. 10th ed. American Association of Cereal Chemistry (AACC), St. Paul, Minnesota, USA.

Benzie I. and Strain J. (1996). The Ferric Reducing Ability of Plasma (FRAP) as a measure of Antioxidant Power: The FRAP Assay. *Analytical Biochemistry*, 239, 70 - 76.

Brand-Williams W., Cuvelier M.E. and Berset C. (1994). Use of a free radical method to evaluate antioxidant activity. *Lebensmittel, Wissenschaft und Technologie*, 28, 25 - 30.

Chesson A. (2006). "Dietary fiber". In: A.M. Stephen, G.O. Phillips & P.A. Williams (Eds.) *Food Polysaccharides and Their Applications*, Second Edition, 629 - 663, CRC Press, USA.

Doublier J.L., Launay B. and Cuvelier G. (1992). "Viscoelastic properties of food gels". In: M.A. Rao & J.F. Steffe (Eds.), *Viscoelastic Properties of Food*, Elsevier Applied Science, NY, USA.

Dreher M. (1999). "Food sources and uses of dietary fiber". In: S.S. Cho, L. Prosky & M. Dreher (Eds.), *Complex Carbohydrates in Foods*, Marcel Dekker Inc., NY, USA.

Dreher M.L. (2001). "Dietary fiber overview". In: S.S. Cho. & M.L. Dreher (Eds.), *Handbook of Dietary Fiber*, Marcel Dekker Inc., NY, USA.

Dubois M., Gilles K.A., Hamilton J.K., Robers P.A. and Smith F. (1956). Colorimetric method for determination of sugars and related substances. *Analytical Chemistry*, 28, 350 - 356.

Endress H.U., Mattes F. and Norz H. (2005). "Pectins" In: Y.H. Hui (Ed.), *Handbook of Food Science Technology and Engineering*, Volume 3, Marcel Dekker, USA.

Fernandez Lopez J., Almela L., Obón J. and Castellar R. (2010). Determination of antioxidant constituents in cactus pear fruits. *Plant Foods for Human Nutrition*, 65, 253 - 259.

Filisetti-Cozzi T.M. and Carpita N.C. (1991). Measurement of uronic acids without interference from neutral sugars. *Analytical Biochemistry*, 197, 157 - 162.

Fissore E.N., Ponce N.M.A., Matkovic L., Stortz C.A, Rojas A.M. and Gerschenson L.N. (2011). Isolation of pectin-enriched products from red beet (*Beta vulgaris* L. var. *conditiva*) wastes: composition and functional properties. *Food Science and Technology International*, 17, 517 - 527.

Fissore E. (2009). Obtención de productos enriquecidos en pectina a partir de residuos de la industrialización de calabaza (*Cucurbita Moschata* Duch Ex Poiret) y remolacha (*Beta Vulgaris* L. var. *conditiva*), y su caracterización. Ph D Thesis - Facultad de Ciencias Exactas y Naturales, Universidad de Buenos Aires. In Spanish.

Fissore E.N., Ponce N.M., Wider E.A., Stortz C.A., Gerschenson L.N. and Rojas A.M. (2009). Commercial cell wall hydrolytic enzymes for producing pectin enriched products from butternut (*Cucurbita moschata* Duchesne ex Poiret). *Journal of Food Engineering*, 93, 293 - 301.

Fissore E.N, Ponce N.M., Stortz C.A., Rojas A.M. and Gerschenson N.L. (2007). Characterisation of fiber obtained from pumpkin (*Cucumis moschata* Duch.) mesocarp through enzymatic treatment. *Food Science and Technology International*, 13, 141 - 151.

Fry S.C. (1986). Cross-linking of matrix polymers in the growing cell walls of angiosperms. *Annual Review of Plant Physiology*, 37, 165 - 186.

Fuentes E., Carle R., Astudillo L., Gúzman L., Gutiérrez M., Carrasco G. and Palomo I. (2013). Antioxidant and antiplatelet activities in extracts from green and fully ripe tomato fruits (*Solanum lycopersicum*) and pomace from industrial tomato processing. *Evidence-Based Complementary and Alternative Medicine*, 1- 9.

Halliwell B. and Gutteridge J.C. (1995). The definition and measurement of antioxidants in biological systems. *Free Radical Biology and Medicine*, 18, 125 - 126.

Jalili T., Medeiros D. and Wildman R. (2007). "Dietary fiber and coronary heart disease". In: R. Wildman (Ed.) *Handbook of Nutraceuticals and Functional Foods*, Second Edition, CRC Press, USA.

Jiménez-Escrig A., Dragsted L.O., Daneshvas B., Pulido R. and Saura-Calixto F. (2003). In Vitro antioxidant activities of edible artichoke (*Cynara scolymus* L.) and effect on biomarkers of antioxidants in rats. *Journal of Agricultural and Food Chemistry*, 51, 5540 - 5545.

Latorre M.E, De Escalada Plá M.F., Rojas A.M. and Gerschenson L.N. (2013). Blanching of red beet (*Beta vulgaris* L. var. *conditiva*) root. Effect of hot water or microwave radiation on cell wall characteristics. *Food Science and Technology*, 50, 193 - 203.

Laufenberg G., Kunz B. and Nystroem M. (2003). Transformation of vegetable waste into value added products: (A) upgrading concept; (B) practical implementations. *Bioresource Technology*, 87, 167 - 198.

Lianda R.L.P., D'Olivera Sant'Ana L., Echeverria A. and Castro R.N. (2012). Antioxidant activity and phenolic composition of Brazilian honeys and their extracts. *Journal of the Brazilian Chemistry Society*, 23, 618 - 627.

Lopes da Silva J.A. and Rao M.A (2006). "Pectins: structure, functionality, and uses". In: A.M. Stephen, G.O. Phillips & P.A. Williams (Eds.), *Food Polysaccharides and Their Applications*, Second Edition, 353 - 411, CRC Press, USA.

Lowry O.H., Rosebrough N.J., Farr A.L. and Randall R.J. (1951). Protein measurement with the Folin phenol reagent. *Journal of Biological Chemistry*, 193, 265 - 275.

Makris D.P., Boskou G. and Andrikopoulos N.K. (2007). Polyphenolic content and in vitro antioxidant characteristics of wine industry and other agri-food solid waste extracts. *Journal of Food Composition and Analysis*, 20, 125 - 132.

Martin-Cabrejas M.A.M., Waldron K.W. and Selvendran R.R. (1994). Cell wall changes in spanish pear during ripening. *Journal of Plant Physiology*, 144, 541 - 548.

Martínez R., Torres P., Meneses M.A., Figueroa J.G., Pérez-Álvarez J.A. and Viuda-Martos M. (2012). Chemical, technological and in vitro antioxidant properties of mango, guava, pineapple and passion fruit dietary fiber concentrate. *Food Chemistry*, 135, 1520 - 1526.

Matos-Chamorro A. and Chambilla-Mamani E. (2010). Importancia de la fibra dietética, sus propiedades funcionales en la alimentación humana y en la industria alimentaria. *Revista de Investigación en Ciencia y Tecnología de Alimentos*, 1, 4 - 17. In Spanish

Meisner N., Muños K., Restovich R., Zapata M.E., Camoletto S., Torrent M.C. and Molinas J. (2011). Fibra Alimentaria: consumo en estudiantes universitarios y asociación con Síndrome de Intestino Irritable. *Invenio*, 14, 91 - 100. In Spanish

Miller Jones, Julie. 2014. CODEX-aligned dietary fiber definitions help to bridge the 'fiber gap'. Nutrition Journal 2014, 13, 34-44.

Naumenko I.V. and Phillipov M.P. (1992). Colorimetric method for determination of acetyl groups in pectic substances. *Akad Nauk Rep Moldova Biol i Khim Nauki*, 1, 56 – 59.

Nawirska A. and Kwasniewska M. (2005). Dietary fiber fractions from fruit and vegetable processing waste. *Food Chemistry*, 91, 221 - 225.

Ng A., Parr A.J., Ingham L.M., Rigby N.M. and Waldron K.M. (1998). Cell wall chemistry of carrots (*Daucus carota* CV. Amstrong) during maturation and storage. *Journal of Agriculture and Food Chemistry*, 46, 2933 - 2939.

Ngouémazong D.E., Tengweh F.F., Fraeye I., Duvetter T., Cardinaels R., Van Loey A., Moldenaers P. and Hendrickx M. (2012). Effect of de-methylesterification on network development and nature of Ca^{2+}-pectin gels: Towards understanding structure-function relations of pectin. *Food Hydrocolloids*, 26, 89 - 98.

Oechslin R., Lutz M.V. and Amadó R. (2003). Pectic substances from apple cellulosic residue: structural characterisation of a new type of rhamnogalacturonan I. *Carbohydrate Polymers,* 51, 301 - 310.

Palafox-Carlos H., Ayala-Zavala J.F. and Gonzáles-Aguilar A. (2011). The role of dietary fiber in the bioaccessibility and bioavailability of fruit and vegetable antioxidants. *Journal of Food Science,* 76, 6 - 15.

Pérez S., Rodríguez-Carvajal M.A. and Doco T. (2003). A complex plant cell wall polysaccharide: rhamnogalacturonan II. A structure in quest of a function. *Biochimie*, 85, 109 - 121.

Pulido R., Bravo L. and Saura-Calixto F. (2000). Antioxidant activity of dietary polyphenols as determined by a modified Ferric Reducing/Antioxidant Power Assay. *Journal of Agricultural and Food Chemistry*, 48, 3396 - 3402.

Saura-Calixto F. (2011). Dietary fiber as a carrier of dietary antioxidants: an essential physiological function. *Journal of Agricultural and Food Chemistry*, 59, 43 - 49.

Selvendran R.R. (1985). Developments in the chemistry and biochemistry of pectic and hemicellulosic polymers. *Journal of Cell Science*, 2, 51 - 88.

Singleton V.L. and Rossi J.A. (1965). Colorimetry of total phenolics with phosphomolybdic – phosphotungstic acid reagents. *American Journal of Enology and Viticulture*, 16, 144 - 158.

Vincken J.P., Schols H.A., Oomen R.J.F.J., McCann M.C., Ulvskov P., Voragen A.G.J. and Visser R.G.F. (2003). If homogalacturonan were a side chain of rhamnogalacturonan I. Implications for cell wall architecture. *Plant Physiology*, 132, 1781 - 1789.

Vu T., Ovarlez G. and Chateau C. (2010). Macroscopic behavior of bidisperse suspensions of noncolloidal particles in yield stress fluids. *Journal of Rheology*, 54, 815 - 833.

Waldron K.W., Ng A., Parker M.L. and Parr A.J. (1997). Ferulic acid dehydrodimers in the cell walls of Beta vulgaris and their possible role in texture. *Journal of the Science of Food and Agriculture*, 74, 2, 221- 228.

Willats W.G.T., Knox J.P. and Mikkelsen J.D. (2006). Pectin: new insights into an old polymer are starting to gel. *Trends in Food Science and Technology*, 17, 97 - 104.

Wood P.J. and Siddiqui I.R. (1971). Determination of methanol and its application for measurement of pectin ester content and pectin methyl esterase activity. *Analytical Biochemistry*, 39, 418 - 428.

Yapo B.M. (2009). Pectin quantity, composition and physicochemical behavior as influenced by the purification process. *Food Research International*, 42, 1197 - 1202.

Yapo B.M. (2011). Pectic substances: From simple pectic polysaccharides to complex pectins - A new hypothetical model. *Carbohydrate Polymers*, 86, 373 - 385.

In: Dietary Fiber
Editor: Marvin E. Clemens
ISBN: 978-1-63463-655-1
© 2015 Nova Science Publishers, Inc.

Chapter 8

DIETARY FIBER INTAKE ASSOCIATED WITH REDUCED RISK OF EPITHELIAL OVARIAN CANCER IN SOUTHERN CHINESE WOMEN

Li Tang, Andy H. Lee**, Dada Su and Colin W. Binns
School of Public Health, Curtin University, Perth, WA, Australia

ABSTRACT

Objective: Ovarian cancer is the third most common gynecological malignancy and the eighth leading cause of cancer-related deaths among women worldwide. The present study aimed to investigate the association between dietary fiber intake and the risk of epithelial ovarian cancer in southern Chinese women.

Methods: A case-control study was undertaken in Guangzhou, Guangdong Province, between 2006 and 2008. Participants were 500 incident ovarian cancer patients and 500 hospital-based controls. Information on habitual foods consumption was obtained by face-to-face interview, from which dietary fiber intakes were estimated using the Chinese food composition tables. Unconditional logistic regression analyses were performed to assess the association between dietary fiber intake and the ovarian cancer risk.

Results: The ovarian cancer patients reported lower intake levels of total dietary fiber and fiber derived from vegetables, fruits and cereals than those of controls. Overall, regular intake of fiber was inversely associated with the ovarian cancer risk, the adjusted odds ratio being 0.09 (95% confidence interval 0.05 to 0.14) for the highest (> 21.9 g) versus the lowest (< 16.5 g) tertile of daily intake, with a significant dose-response relationship ($p < 0.001$). Similar reduction in risk was also apparent for high intake level of vegetable fiber, but to a lesser extent for fruit fiber and cereal fiber.

Conclusion: Habitual intake of dietary fiber was inversely associated with the incidence of epithelial ovarian cancer in southern Chinese women.

Keywords: Ovarian cancer; case-control study; dietary fiber; China

* Corresponding author: Professor Andy H. Lee, School of Public Health, Curtin University, GPO Box U 1987, Perth, WA, 6845, Australia, Phone: +61-8-92664180, Fax: +61-8-92662958, Email: Andy.Lee@curtin.edu.au

INTRODUCTION

Ovarian cancer is the third most common gynecological malignancy and has the eighth highest mortality rate of all cancers in women worldwide [1]. In 2012, more than 238,700 new cases were diagnosed, with an estimated 151,900 women died from this cancer [1]. Approximately 90% of ovarian malignancies are epithelial in origin [2]. Ovarian cancer is generally diagnosed at an advanced stage, as the symptoms are vague and non-specific [3]. Exploring ways to prevent this disease is therefore important.

Earlier research has suggested a possible protective effect of dietary fiber against the development of ovarian cancer. A population-based case-control study undertaken in the USA reported a 57% risk reduction for women with the highest intake of dietary fiber [4]. Similarly, a case-control study conducted in Hangzhou, China, showed a significant inverse association between the ovarian cancer risk and intake of dietary fiber [5]. However, little association was found between intake of fiber and overall ovarian cancer risk in a prospective population-based cohort study from Sweden. Dietary fiber was marginally inversely associated with risk of borderline ovarian cancer in the cohort, but not with risk of invasive ovarian cancer [6].

A recently published report from the World Cancer Research Fund (WCRF) indicated that the evidence for an association between dietary fiber and the risk of ovarian cancer was either too limited or inconsistent for a conclusion [7]. Furthermore, only a few studies have investigated intakes of specific sources of fiber in relation to ovarian cancer risk [6, 8]. The primary sources of dietary fiber are vegetables, fruits and cereals. In view of the inconclusive epidemiological evidence, the present study aimed to assess the relationship between dietary fiber intake and the risk of epithelial ovarian cancer among southern Chinese women.

METHODS

Study Design and Subjects

A hospital-based case-control study was conducted in Guangzhou, the capital city of Guangdong Province of southern China, between August 2006 and July 2008. Subjects were recruited from four public hospitals, namely, The Overseas Hospital (affiliated with Jinan University), Zhujiang Hospital, General Hospital of Guangzhou Military Command, and Second Affiliated Hospital of Zhongshan University. To be eligible, all subjects were required to be under 75 years of age and have resided in the metropolitan Guangzhou area for at least the past ten years.

Medical records and pathology reports were reviewed to identify patients newly diagnosed with ovarian cancer within the past 12 months. Pathological diagnoses were based on the International Histological Classification of Ovarian Tumors [9]. Patients were excluded when ovarian cancer was histopathologically confirmed to be neither the primary nor final diagnosis, over 75 years of age, or if they had self-reported memory problems affecting their recall of past events. Of the total 504 patients identified, 500 consented to participate.

Meanwhile, controls were recruited from inpatients at the same hospitals from Ophthalmology, Orthopaedics, Respiratory Diseases, Gastroenterology and Physiotherapy departments. Exclusion criteria for controls were previous diagnosis of malignant disease; history of bilateral oophorectomy; having self-reported memory problems; on long-term medical diet; in addition to non-residency and age above 75 years. Whenever more controls were available than could be interviewed, the final selection was made using random numbers generated from the software Research Randomizer (http://www.socialpsychology.org). Of the 512 eligible controls recruited to frequency matched with cases by age (± 5 years), 500 women eventually gave their consent to be interviewed. There were no significant differences in age, education level and marital status between participants and non-participants.

The study was approved by the participating hospitals and the Human Research Ethics Committee of Curtin University (number HR 78/2006). Written informed consent was obtained from all participants. They were assured of the right to withdraw any time without prejudice.

Data Collection

All participants were interviewed by trained interviewers in either Mandarin or Cantonese, usually in the presence of their next-of-kin to help the recall of dietary habits. Both participants and interviewers were blinded to the study hypothesis.

The structured questionnaire comprised sections on demographic characteristics, anthropometry, reproductive history, hormonal status, past and family medical history, diet and personal habits such as cigarette smoking and alcohol consumption. Current weight, weight five years before the interview and height were used to calculate body mass index (BMI) at both times. Self-reported data were cross-checked with medical records whenever possible.

Participants were also requested to estimate the average time they had engaged in physical activities using a validated questionnaire [10].

Intensity was classified by the amount of energy or effort a person expends in performing the activity. Physical activity at each intensity level was quantified in terms of metabolic equivalent tasks (MET) hours per week, with intensity codes 7.5, 6.0 and 4.5 MET assigned to strenuous sports, vigorous work and moderate activity, respectively. Total physical activity was then calculated by summing the product of MET score and activity duration over the three intensity levels.

Information on dietary habits was collected using a 125-item semi-quantitative food frequency questionnaire, which had been validated and included cereals, fruits and vegetables commonly consumed in southern China [11, 12]. Frequency and amount of intake were recorded in detail.

The reference recall period for dietary variables was five years before diagnosis for cases and five years before interview for controls. For each individual, daily intakes (g) of dietary fiber from vegetables, fruits and cereals were estimated using the Chinese food composition tables [13].

Total energy intake (kcal) was calculated in a similar manner, based on the energy content of each food or beverage item and the amount consumed.

Statistical Analysis

Descriptive statistics were used to compare the sample characteristics between case and control groups. Unconditional logistic regression analyses were then performed to ascertain the effects of dietary fiber intakes on the epithelial ovarian cancer risk. For each exposure variable of interest, the tertiles of consumption among controls were obtained, with the lowest level being the reference category.

In addition to reporting crude and adjusted odds ratios (OR) and corresponding 95% confidence intervals (CI), dose-response relationships were assessed by tests for linear trend. Confounding variables included in the logistic regression models were age at interview (years, continuous), education level (none or primary, secondary, vocational or tertiary), BMI (5 years ago, kg/m^2, continuous), physical activity (MET-hours/week, continuous), fresh meat consumption (g/day, continuous), seafood consumption (g/day, continuous), total energy intake (kcal/day, continuous), parity (continuous), oral contraceptive use (never, ever), menopausal status (pre, post), tubal ligation (no, yes), history of hormone replacement therapy (no, yes), smoking status (never, past, current), alcohol drinking (no, yes), and family history of ovarian or breast cancer in first-degree relatives (no, yes). Participants who consumed at least 500 ml of alcoholic beverages per week were classified as 'yes', otherwise they were referred to as 'no'. These variables were either established or plausible risk factors from the literature. Sensitivity of the analyses to histologic subtypes of epithelial ovarian tumors was also conducted. All statistical analyses were performed using the SPSS package version 20.0 (IBM, Armonk, NY, USA).

RESULTS

Half of the 500 epithelial ovarian cancer patients were histologically diagnosed as serous carcinoma, while mucinous tumors comprised 16% of the cases. Other histologic subtypes included borderline malignancy (13.1%), undifferentiated carcinoma (11.8%), endometrioid cystadenocarcinoma (3.8%), mixed epithelial cystadenocarcinoma (2.6%), clear cell carcinoma (1.4%), transitional cell carcinoma (0.8%) and malignant Brenner's tumor (0.6%).

Table 1 summarizes characteristics of the sample by case-control status. The participants were on average 59.4 (SD 6.1) years old. They were predominantly post-menopausal (95.2%). Most of them had attained secondary school education or above (59.9%), never had a tubal ligation (64.9%), were non-smokers (96.6%) and seldom drank alcoholic beverages (72.4%). Women with ovarian cancer tended to have less oral contraceptive use and lower parities, higher mean BMI, consume significantly less seafood and were less physically active than controls. With respect to dietary fiber, the cases had significantly lower daily intakes of total fiber and fiber derived from vegetables, fruits and cereals than their control counterparts (Table 2).

Table 3 presents the logistic regression results. Total fiber intake was significantly inversely associated with risk of epithelial ovarian cancer, with a significant dose-response relationship (p for trend < 0.001). The adjusted OR was 0.09 (95% CI: 0.05 to 0.14) for women whose total intake exceeded 21.9 g/day relative to those less than 16.5 g/day.

Table 1. Characteristics of participants by case-control status for southern Chinese women

Variable	Cases n (%)	Controls n (%)	p [a]
Marital status			0.83
Never married	7 (1.4%)	8 (1.6%)	
Married	449 (89.8%)	443 (88.6%)	
Widowed or divorced or separated	44 (8.8%)	49 (9.8%)	
Education level			0.90
None or primary	204 (40.8%)	197 (39.4%)	
Secondary	171 (34.2%)	175 (35.0%)	
Vocational or tertiary	125 (25.0%)	128 (25.6%)	
Parity			< 0.01
0	8 (1.6%)	14 (2.8%)	
1	172 (34.4%)	143 (28.6%)	
2	219 (43.8%)	176 (35.2%)	
≥ 3	101 (20.2%)	167 (33.4%)	
Oral contraceptive use			< 0.01
Never	417 (83.4%)	380 (76.0%)	
Ever	83 (16.6%)	120 (24.0%)	
Menopausal status			0.24
Pre	28 (5.6%)	20 (4.0%)	
Post	472 (94.4%)	480 (96.0%)	
Tubal ligation			0.95
No	325 (65.0%)	324 (64.8%)	
Yes	175 (35.0%)	176 (35.2%)	
Hormone replacement therapy			1.00
No	493 (98.6%)	493 (98.6%)	
Yes	7 (1.4%)	7 (1.4%)	
Smoking status			0.37
Never	481 (96.2%)	485 (97.0%)	
Past	14 (2.8%)	8 (1.6%)	
Current	5 (1.0%)	7 (1.4%)	
Alcohol drinking			0.16
No	352 (70.4%)	372 (74.4%)	
Yes	148 (29.6%)	128 (25.6%)	
Family history of ovarian or breast cancer in first-degree relatives			0.39
No	480 (96.0%)	485 (97.0%)	
Yes	20 (4.0%)	15 (3.0%)	
	mean (SD)	mean (SD)	
Age at interview (years)	59.1 (5.7)	59.7 (6.5)	0.10
Body mass index (5 years ago, kg/m^2)	21.7 (2.5)	21.1 (2.3)	< 0.01
Physical activity (MET-hours/week)	16.2 (14.1)	18.8 (13.0)	< 0.01
Fresh meat consumption (g/day)	288 (157.9)	285 (166.9)	0.74
Seafood consumption (g/day)	122 (74.0)	141 (136.6)	< 0.01

[a] Chi-square or Student's t-test for difference between cases and controls

Table 2. Comparison of dietary fiber intake between case and control groups among southern Chinese women

Daily intake (g)	Cases mean (SD)	Controls mean (SD)	p [a]
Total dietary fiber	14.8 (4.8)	22.2 (14.9)	< 0.001
Vegetable fiber	6.8 (2.7)	11.1 (8.0)	< 0.001
Fruit fiber	4.9 (2.7)	7.2 (7.6)	< 0.001
Cereal fiber	3.2 (1.7)	3.8 (2.8)	< 0.001

[a] Student's t-test for mean difference between cases and controls.

Table 3. Crude and adjusted odds ratios (95% confidence intervals) of ovarian cancer risk for dietary fiber intake among southern Chinese women

Daily intake (g)	Cases n (%)	Controls n (%)	Crude OR (95% CI)	Adjusted OR [a] (95% CI)	p for trend [a]
Total dietary fiber					
< 16.5	357 (71.4%)	168 (33.6%)	1.00	1.00	< 0.001
16.5 – 21.9	112 (22.4%)	167 (33.4%)	0.32 (0.23, 0.43)	0.33 (0.24, 0.46)	
> 21.9	31 (6.2%)	165 (33.0%)	0.09 (0.06, 0.14)	0.09 (0.05, 0.14)	
Vegetable fiber					< 0.001
< 8.2	392 (78.4%)	171 (34.2%)	1.00	1.00	
8.2 – 10.9	78 (15.6%)	159 (31.8%)	0.21 (0.16, 0.30)	0.22 (0.16, 0.31)	
> 10.9	30 (6.0%)	170 (34.0%)	0.08 (0.05, 0.12)	0.08 (0.05, 0.13)	
Fruit fiber					< 0.001
< 4.4	252 (50.4%)	166 (33.2%)	1.00	1.00	
4.4 – 6.9	166 (33.2%)	171 (34.2%)	0.64 (0.48, 0.85)	0.66 (0.48, 0.90)	
> 6.9	82 (16.4%)	163 (32.6%)	0.33 (0.24, 0.46)	0.38 (0.27, 0.54)	
Cereal fiber					0.211
< 2.6	235 (47.0%)	170 (34.0%)	1.00	1.00	
2.6 – 3.9	163 (32.6%)	170 (34.0%)	0.69 (0.52, 0.93)	0.76 (0.56, 1.04)	
> 3.9	102 (20.4%)	160 (32.0%)	0.46 (0.34, 0.63)	0.61 (0.43, 0.88)	

[a] From separate logistic regression models adjusting for age at interview (years, continuous), education level (none or primary, secondary, vocational or tertiary), body mass index (5 years ago, kg/m^2, continuous), physical activity (MET-hours/week, continuous), fresh meat consumption (g/day, continuous), seafood consumption (g/day, continuous), total energy intake (kcal/day, continuous), parity (continuous), oral contraceptive use (never, ever), menopausal status (pre, post), tubal ligation (no, yes), hormone replacement therapy (no, yes), smoking status (never, past, current), alcohol drinking (no, yes), and family history of ovarian or breast cancer in first-degree relatives (no, yes).

Significant reduction in cancer risk was also found for high intake of vegetable fiber, but to a lesser extent for fruit fiber and cereal fiber. There was no significant dose-response relationship between cereal fiber intake and risk of epithelial ovarian cancer (p for trend = 0.211). Further subgroup analysis for serous and mucinous ovarian tumors produced similar results which were omitted for brevity. Analyses were not performed for other histologic subtypes due to the low number of cases available.

Discussion

This case-control study of southern Chinese women suggested a protective role for dietary fiber intake against epithelial ovarian cancer. Our results are in line with those of previous case-control studies conducted in China [5] and in the USA [4, 14], but different from a Canadian case-control study [15]. With reference to the source of fiber, our findings are somewhat consistent with an Italian case-control study, which also found an inverse association between vegetable fiber intake and ovarian cancer risk, but no associations were evident for fruit fiber or cereal fiber intake [8]. On the other hand, no apparent association was observed between intake of total dietary fiber, vegetable or cereal fiber and ovarian cancer risk in a Swedish longitudinal study [6]. Differences between populations in fruit, vegetable and cereal consumption levels may partly explain the conflicting epidemiological findings [8].

Several biologically plausible mechanisms may explain the preventive effect of dietary fiber on ovarian cancer risk. Dietary fiber may influence ovarian carcinogenesis by reducing the bioavailability of steroid hormones via changes in bacterial macroflora, lowering serum levels and availability of oestrogens, and increasing protection of lignans or other phytoestrogens [8]. Dietary fiber is also known to be associated with reduced glycaemic load and improved insulin sensitivity [16], favourably influencing insulin-like growth factor 1 (IGF-1), which is a promoter of the progression of carcinogenesis at various sites including the ovary [17]. Moreover, high-fiber foods typically contain antioxidants and phytochemicals with potentially inhibitory effects on the process of carcinogenesis [18].

In this study, a standardized identification procedure had been implemented that ensured the ascertainment of cases was maximised and complete. To avoid misclassification of the case-control status, we recruited only incident patients who had been diagnosed with ovarian cancer within the past 12 months and subsequently confirmed with pathology. All controls were carefully screened. In addition, habitual food consumption was measured using a validated and reliable questionnaire specifically developed for the southern Chinese population, with information on frequency and quantity of intake recorded in detail. To determine the effect of dietary fiber intake, information on other exposures and confounding factors such as physical activity, tobacco smoking and alcohol drinking was also collected. It was possible that some ovarian cancer patients might have modified their dietary behaviors since the onset of the disease. Therefore, the reference period for the dietary recall was set at five years before diagnosis to avoid reverse causation.

A major limitation concerns the inherent retrospective cross-sectional design so that any cause-effect relationship between dietary fiber intake and ovarian cancer risk could not be established. Selection bias was unavoidable because all participants were voluntary and the hospital-based controls were not randomly selected from the community. Nevertheless, the four participating hospitals serve the entire catchment region so that our subjects were still representative of the target population. Recruitment bias was also minimized by sampling from different hospitals. Although the recall of habitual vegetable, fruit and cereal consumption should not be affected by the case-control status, dietary assessment was made based on self-report, which probably introduced some recall error in the participant response. Therefore, face-to-face interviews were conducted in the presence of their next-of-kin to help memory recall and to improve the accuracy of their answers [19]. Information bias and recall bias were unlikely because the nurses who conducted the interview and all participants were blind to the study hypothesis, while the potential protective effect of dietary fiber against ovarian cancer has not been established in southern China at the time of interview. Finally, residual confounding might still exist even though established risk factors have been controlled for in the multivariable logistic regression models.

CONCLUSION

Habitual intake of dietary fiber was inversely associated with the risk of epithelial ovarian cancer in southern China, with significant dose-response relationships observed for total fiber and fire derived from vegetables and fruits. While further prospective cohort studies are required to confirm the findings, the consumption of high-fiber foods may offer protection and enhance the survival of this deadly disease.

ACKNOWLEDGMENTS

The authors are indebted to the ovarian cancer patients and control participants who agreed to be interviewed. Thanks are also due to the medical and nursing staff of the participating hospitals for their assistance in patient recruitment.

Conflict of Interest

No potential conflicts of interest for all authors.

REFERENCES

[1] Ferlay J, Soerjomataram I, Ervik M, Dikshit R, Eser S, Mathers C, et al. GLOBOCAN 2012 v1.0, Cancer Incidence and Mortality Worldwide: IARC CancerBase No. 11. Lyon, France: *International Agency for Research on Cancer;* 2013.

[2] Cho KR, Shih Ie M. Ovarian cancer. *Annu. Rev. Pathol*. 2009;4:287-313.

[3] Lutz AM, Willmann JK, Drescher CW, Ray P, Cochran FV, Urban N, et al. Early diagnosis of ovarian carcinoma: is a solution in sight? *Radiology*. 2011;259(2):329-45.

[4] McCann SE, Freudenheim JL, Marshall JR, Graham S. Risk of human ovarian cancer is related to dietary intake of selected nutrients, phytochemicals and food groups. *J. Nutr.* 2003;133(6):1937-42.

[5] Zhang M, Lee AH, Binns CW. Reproductive and dietary risk factors for epithelial ovarian cancer in China. *Gynecol. Oncol.* 2004;92(1):320-6.
[6] Hedelin M, Lof M, Andersson TM, Adlercreutz H, Weiderpass E. Dietary phytoestrogens and the risk of ovarian cancer in the women's lifestyle and health cohort study. *Cancer Epidemiol. Biomarkers Prev.* 2011;20(2):308-17.
[7] World Cancer Research Fund/American Institute for Cancer Research. Continuous Update Project Report. Food, Nutrition, Physical Activity, and the Prevention of Ovarian Cancer 2014. Washington, DC, USA: AICR; 2014.
[8] Pelucchi C, La Vecchia C, Chatenoud L, Negri E, Conti E, Montella M, et al. Dietary fibres and ovarian cancer risk. *Eur. J. Cancer.* 2001;37(17):2235-9.
[9] Heintz AP, Odicino F, Maisonneuve P, Quinn MA, Benedet JL, Creasman WT, et al. Carcinoma of the ovary. FIGO 26th Annual Report on the Results of Treatment in Gynecological Cancer. *Int. J. Gynaecol. Obstet.* 2006;95 Suppl 1:S161-92.
[10] Lee AH, Su D, Pasalich M, Wong YL, Binns CW. Habitual physical activity reduces risk of ovarian cancer: a case-control study in southern *China. Prev. Med.* 2013;57 Suppl:S31-3.
[11] Ke L, Toshiro T, Fengyan S, Ping Y, Xiaoling D, Kazuo T. Relative validity of a semi-quantitative food frequency questionnaire versus 3 day weighed diet records in middle-aged inhabitants in Chaoshan area, China. *Asian Pac. J. Cancer Prev.* 2005;6(3):376-81.
[12] Song FY, Toshiro T, Li K, Yu P, Lin XK, Yang HL, et al. Development of a semi-quantitative food frequency questionnaire for middle-aged inhabitants in the Chaoshan area, China. *World J. Gastroenterol.* 2005;11(26):4078-84.
[13] Chinese Center for Disease Control and Prevention. China Food Composition Table. 2nd ed. Beijing, China: Peking University Medical Press; 2009.
[14] McCann SE, Moysich KB, Mettlin C. Intakes of selected nutrients and food groups and risk of ovarian cancer. *Nutr. Cancer.* 2001;39(1):19-28.
[15] Pan SY, Ugnat AM, Mao Y, Wen SW, Johnson KC. A case-control study of diet and the risk of ovarian cancer. *Cancer Epidemiol. Biomarkers Prev.* 2004 Sep;13(9):1521-7.
[16] Schulze MB, Liu S, Rimm EB, Manson JE, Willett WC, Hu FB. Glycemic index, glycemic load, and dietary fiber intake and incidence of type 2 diabetes in younger and middle-aged women. *Am. J. Clin. Nutr.* 2004;80(2):348-56.
[17] Brokaw J, Katsaros D, Wiley A, Lu L, Su D, Sochirca O, et al. IGF-I in epithelial ovarian cancer and its role in disease progression. *Growth Factors.* 2007;25(5):346-54.
[18] Murdoch WJ, Martinchick JF. Oxidative damage to DNA of ovarian surface epithelial cells affected by ovulation: carcinogenic implication and chemoprevention. *Exp. Biol. Med.* (Maywood). 2004;229(6):546-52.
[19] Liang W, Binns C, Lee AH, Huang R, Hu D. The reliability of dietary and lifestyle information obtained from spouses in an elderly Chinese population. *Asia Pac. J. Public Health.* 2008;20(2):87-93.

In: Dietary Fiber
Editor: Marvin E. Clemens

ISBN: 978-1-63463-655-1
© 2015 Nova Science Publishers, Inc.

Chapter 9

Dietary Fiber From Agroindustrial By-Products: Orange Peel Flour As Functional Ingredient in Meat Products

M. Lourdes Pérez-Chabela, [1,*] ***Juana Chaparro-Hernández*** [1] ***and Alfonso Totosaus*** [2]

[1]Biotechnology Department, Universidad Autónoma Metropolitana Iztapalapa, Distrito Federal, México City, México

[2]Food Science Lab/Pilot plant, Tecnológico Estudios Superiores Ecatepec, Estado de México, Ecatepec, México

Abstract

Recently, the use of alternative fiber sources obtained from agroindustrial sub-products as fruit peels. Meat extenders comprise material that improve water retention (yield) and texture in cooked meat products. The most employed are potato starch and kappa carrageenan. The interaction of these three ingredients in a cooked sausage formulation was studied by means of a mixture design approach. Fiber in orange peel flour increased moisture and water retention, besides decreased oxidative rancidity in cooked sausages. Orange peel flour reduced sausages luminosity and redness, increasing yellowness. Fiber contained in orange peel flour improving texture resulting in softer but more cohesive and resilient sausages. Cooked meat products conditions (temperature and ionic strength) affected the functionality of meat extenders like potato starch and carrageenan. This indicates that orange peel flour as a cheap and viable fiber source can replace more expensive meat extenders, as potato starch or carrageenan.

* Corresponding author. Tel.: +52 55 58044717. E-mail address: lpch@xanum.uam.mx.

INTRODUCTION

The additives more employed in sausages manufacture as fillers (non-meat ingredients with substantially high carbohydrate content) are starches and gums, like carrageenan. Starches are employed as water binders to increase yield, reduce cooking loses, improve texture and enhance water and fat retention. Potato starch is the most employed in the meat industry since its lower gelatinization temperature allows a higher water holding capacity at sausages processing conditions (Zhang and Barbut, 2005; Kerry and Kerry, 2006). Carrageenan in meat products contributes to gel formation enhancing water retention to improve texture and product juiciness (Trius et al., 1996). On other hand, sub-products generated by fruit processing industry to elaborate juices are a source of dietetic fiber that can be employed as food ingredient (Larioet al., 2004). Considering the orange, for example, where approximately 50% of the fruit is discarded after juice pressing and the total phenolic compounds content is 15% higher in the peel that in juice because the albedo and flavedo content (Escobedo-Avellaneda et al., 2013). Citrus fibers are a better alternative to cereal fibers since the content of soluble dietetic fiber and bioactive associated compounds (flavonoids, polyphenols, caroteinoids, and vitamin C) (Balasundramet al., 2006; Vermaet al., 2010; Moraes-Crizel et al., 2013). The use of these relatively new fiber sources from agro-industrial sub-products as dietetic fiber in meat products could make them more attractive to consumers (Mehta et al., 2013).

The objective of this work was to determinate the effect of orange peel flour, potato starch and carrageenan, employing a mixture design approach, on physicochemical and textural properties of sausages elaborated with mechanically deboned poultry.

MATERIALS AND METHODS

Orange Peel Flour

Orange peel flour was elaborated from pressed oranges recollected in the East side of Mexico City. In 2012, orange production in Mexico was 3,666,790 ton, representing the 5.9% of the world production. Orange is mainly consumed internally in fresh (85-90%) for juice elaboration, and around 1% is processed as pasteurized juice (SIAP, 2013). Peels were collected and transported in plastic boxes, washed in cold tap water and stored under refrigeration (5±1 °C) until processing. Fruit peels were equilibrated at room temperature for 2 h before being cut into small cubic pieces and dried at 60 °C for approximately 24 h in an air convection oven (Craft Instrumentos Científicos, México City, México). Dried peels were ground in a mill and sieved consecutively with mesh sizes 100, 80, 50 and 20 to obtain a regular and homogeneous powder called flour.

Orange peel was analyzed determining the percent of ashes (AOAC Official Method 940.26), ethereal extract (AOAC Official Method 991.36), total protein by Kjeldhal method (AOAC Official Method 920.53), and total fiber (AOAC Official Method 991.43) (AOAC, 1999).

Sausages Elaboration

For sausage elaboration mechanically deboned poultry meat (Tyson de México, Torreón, México) was employed. Frozen mechanically deboned poultry meat (56%, w/w) was grounded in a Moulinex DPA2 Food Processor (Moulinex, Ecully, France), mixing with salt (2.10%, w/w), Hamine® phosphates mixture (McCormick-Pesa, México City, México, 0.18% w/w), curing salt (0.03% w/w) and the half of ice until obtain a homogeneous paste. Frozen pork back fat (5%, w/w) was incorporated and the non-meat ingredients (orange peel flour, potato starch and carrageenan) were mixed in the paste with the rest of ice. Non-meat ingredients proportions are listed in Table 1. Meat batters from the different formulation were stuffed in 2 cm diameter cellulose casing, cooked in water bath until internal temperature reached 72 °C (around 15 minutes), ice cooled and vacuum packed until analysis. A total of two batches (1 kg) of each formulation were elaborated.

Table 1. Non-meat extenders proportions employed in the experimental design

Mixture	Orange peelflour		Potatostarch		Carrageenan	
	Proportion	%	Proportion	%	Proportion	%
1	0.00	0.00	0.00	0.00	1.00	1.00
2	0.00	0.00	0.50	2.50	0.50	050
3	0.17	0.43	0.66	3.30	0.17	0.17
4	0.00	0.00	1.00	5.00	0.00	0.00
5	0.17	0.43	0.17	0.85	0.66	0.66
6	0.33	0.83	0.34	0.67	0.33	0.34
7	0.50	1.25	0.00	0.00	0.50	0.50
8	0.66	1.65	0.17	0.85	0.17	0.17
9	0.50	1.25	0.50	2.50	0.00	0.00
10	1.00	2.50	0.00	0.00	0.00	0.00

Total Moisture, Expressible Moisture and Oxidative Rancidity Determination

Moisture content was determined according AOAC Official Method No. 950.46 (AOAC, 1999). Two g of sample was placed in an aluminum capsule at constant weight and heated in an oven at 110 °C for 12 h. Samples were then removed and the percentage of moisture was calculated based on weight difference. Expressible moisture was determined adapting the methodology reported by Jauregui et al. (1981). Three pieces of Whatman #4 filter paper were weighted, folded in a thimble shape with 2±0.3 g of ground meat batter sample and centrifuged at 3000 × g during 20 min at 4°C. Expressible moisture was reported as the percent weight lost from the original sample.

Oxidative rancidity was determinate using the methodology modified by Zipser and Watts (1962). Ten g of grounded sample was mixed with 49 mL of distilled water at 50 °C, adding one mL of sulfanilamide-HCl solution (0.5% and 20%, respectively, v/v). Subsequently, the sample was transferred to a 500 mL Erlenmeyer flask containing 48 mL of distilled water at 50 °C and 2 mL of HCl solution (50% v/v), plus 2 drops of silicone based antifoam. The contents of the flask was distilled about 10-15 minutes or until obtain 50 mL of distillate. An aliquot of 5 mL was taken and mixed with 5 mL of thiobarbituric acid solution (0.02M in glacial acetic acid 90%). Samples were placed in boiling water for 35 minutes, cooled and the absorbance was measured at 538 nm. The concentration of malonaldehyde (mg/kg of sample) was calculated extrapolating the absorbance against a 1, 1, 3, 3-tetraethoxypropane (3×10^{-3} g/L) solution, according to the report by Lawlor et al. (2000).

Texture Profile Analysis

Textural properties were evaluated via a texture profile analysis in a TAXT2i (Texture Technologies Corporation, Scarsdale, NY, USA; Stable Micro Systems, Godalming, UK), equipped with a 5 kg load cell and a 25-mm diameter acrylic probe. Sausage samples were cut in 20-mm length cylinders and axially compressed the half of their original height in two consecutive cycles, at a constant cross-head speed of 1 mm/s with a waiting period of 5 s. From the force-deformation curves textural profile parameters were calculated as: hardness (maximum force detected during compression), cohesiveness (internal bond strength that give structure to the sample) and resilience (energy stored in the sample that allows you to recover to some extent its original form) (Szczceniak, 1963; Bourne, 1978).

Experimental Design and Data Analysis

A three component constrained simplex lattice mixture design was employed. Mixtures components was three non-meat extenders, as carrageenan (Fabpsa FX6 kappa carragenaan, Fabpsa SA de CV, Mexico City) (X_1), potato starch (KMC Ingredients, Brande, Denmark); (X_2) and orange peel flour (X_3). Components were expressed as fractions of the mixture and the sum ($X_1+X_2+X_3$) of the proportions was one. The ten points consisted of three single ingredients systems, three two-ingredients mixtures and four thee-ingredient mixtures (Figure 1). Scheffe's canonical special cubic equation for 3 components was fitted to data collected at each experimental point using backward stepwise multiple regression analysis as described by Cornell (1980). This canonical model differs from full polynomial models in that it does not contain a constant term, i.e., it has a zero intercept. Variables in the regression models, which represent two-ingredient or three-ingredient interaction terms, were referred to as "non-linear" terms. Canonical special cubic equation postulated was:

$$\eta=\beta_1X_1+\beta_2X_2+\beta_3X_3+\beta_{12}X_1X_2+\beta_{13}X_1X_3+\beta_{23}X_2X_3+\beta_{123}X_1X_2X_3$$

where η is a predictive dependent variable (total moisture, expressible moisture, oxidative rancidity, CIE-Lab color, texture profile analysis); β_1, β_2, β_3, β_{12}, β_{13}, β_{23} and β_{123} are the corresponding parameters estimates for each linear and cross-product term produced for the prediction models or carrageenan (X_1), potato starch (X_2), and orange peel flour (X_3). Data were analyzed in SAS statistical package version 8.0 (SAS Institute, Cary, North Carolina) with the ADX interface, experimental designs, mixtures.

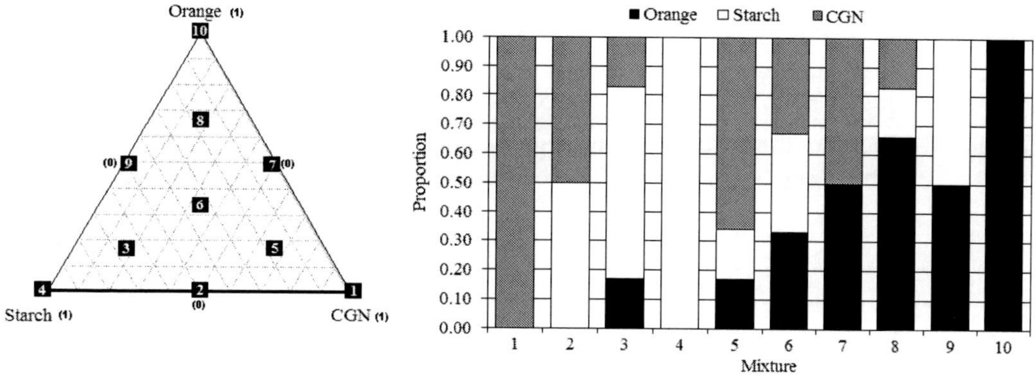

Figure 1. Three components simple centroid design.

RESULTS AND DISCUSSION

Total Moisture, Expressible Moisture and Oxidative Rancidity

Composition of the orange peel flour was: 5.40±0.25% ethereal extract, 3.53±0.53% protein, 6.15±0.05% ashes and 38.11±0.56% total fiber.

For total moisture, the three mixtures components presented a significantly higher effect ($p<0.01$) on this property (Table 2). In regression equation ($R^2= 82.18$), the three parameters had similar values. This means that non-meat extenders water retention was similar in meat batters during and after thermal process. In the isoresponse curve (Figure 2a) potato starch presented a constant effect since isoresponse lines were perpendicular to this vertex. Nonetheless, higher moisture values were obtained close to carrageenan or orange peel vertexes (pure components). For expressible moisture, the three mixture design components had a significantly higher ($p<0.01$) effect on the sausages capacity to retain water. According to regression equation ($R^2= 81.50$), orange peel flour had lower influence (lower released water values) on expressible moisture, whereas potato starch and carrageenan increased water release (Table 2). This was reflected on isoresponse curve, where the carrageenan and potato starch vertexes had higher expressible moisture values (Figure 2b). In this view, at higher orange peel flour proportions, at the employed experimental conditions, the expressible moisture (ability of a system to hold water present in excess and under the influence of an external force) decreased with a concomitant increase in total moisture, as compared to potato starch or carrageenan.

Hydration properties of different meat extenders depend on their characteristics. Carrageenan and orange peel flour increased sausages moisture. In sausages elaborated with mechanically deboned meat, it has been reported that the use of carrageenan increased the water holding capacity, since carrageenan was placed in the interstitial spaces in the protein network, decreasing the compaction of the gel network, allowing bind more water (Ayadi*et al.*, 2009). In same manner, moisture and water retention was improved when potato starch was employed in sausages formulation (Dzieszuk et al., 2005; Liu et al., 2008).

Nonetheless, lower moisture was retained by starch since their hydration depends on the starch granule gelatinization (Murphy, 2000). Higher moistures values were detected at higher orange peel flour proportions, because the higher fiber content.

Table 2. Regression model and Analysis of Variance for the total moisture, expressible moisture and oxidative rancidity of the different formulated sausages

Total moisture (%)= 65.12 Orange peel +62.59 Starch +65.72 CGN, R^2= 82.18					
Source	DF	SS	MS	F	Pr>F
Orange peel	1	7744.845	7744.645	2205.112	0.0001
Starch	1	7156.883	7156.883	2037.721	0.0001
CGN	1	7891.932	7891.932	2247.004	0.0001
Model	2	8.197	4.098	1.167	0.3652
Error	7	24.585	3.512		
Total	9	32.782			
Expressible moisture (%)= 12.42 Orange peel +16.59 Starch +18.93 CGN, R^2= 81.50					
Source	DF	SS	MS	F	Pr>F
Orange peel	1	281.828	281.828	61.884	0.0001
Starch	1	503.266	503.266	110.514	0.0001
CGN	1	655.115	655.115	143.854	0.0001
Model	2	32.472	16.235	3.565	0.0455
Error	7	31.879	4.554		
Total	9	64.356			
Oxidative rancidity (mg MLD/kg)= 0.1408 Orange peel +0.5629 Starch +0.4772 CGN – 0.9839 Orange peel*Starch, R^2= 92.69					
Source	DF	SS	MS	F	Pr>F
Orange peel	1	0.0268	0.0268	2.841	0.0392
Starch	1	0.4291	0.4291	45.769	0.0012
CGN	1	0.4137	0.4137	44.127	0.0072
Orange peel*Starch	1	0.0495	0.0495	5.247	0.0383
Model	3	0.2367	0.7891	8.417	0.0216
Error	4	0.0562	0.0093		
Total	9	0.2929			

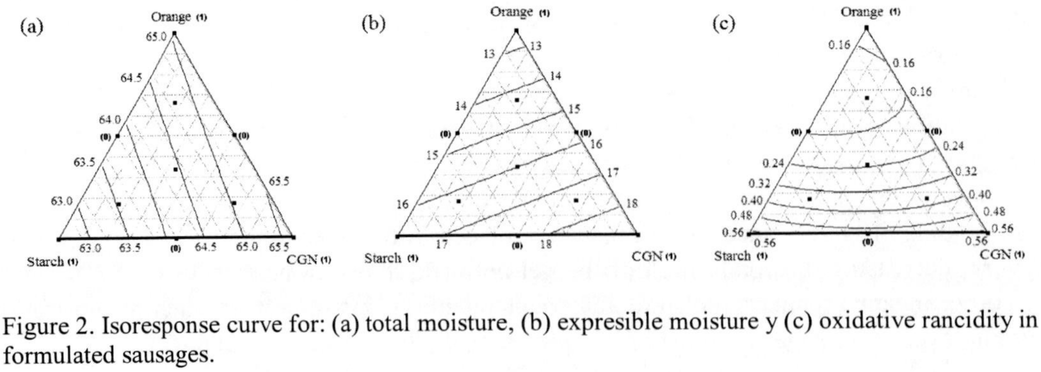

Figure 2. Isoresponse curve for: (a) total moisture, (b) expresible moisture y (c) oxidative rancidity in formulated sausages.

Fiber application in meat products help to retain water and decrease cooking loses since fiber inclusion contributes to bind water and keep product juiciness (Verma et al., 2010; Yalinkiliç et al., 2012). Carrageenan or fiber contained in orange peel flour hydrated more easily than starch, increasing total moisture and retaining more water into the meat system.

Sausages oxidative rancidity was significantly ($p<0.05$) affected by the components in mixture design. Carrageenan and potato starch had a significantly higher ($p<0.01$) effect on this parameter, where according to regression equation (R^2= 92.69) carrageenan and potato starch increased the lipid oxidation in sausages, while orange peel flour decreased lipid oxidation (negative sign in equation). In same manner, interaction between orange peel flour and potato starch also decreased the rancidity values (Table 2). In the isoresponse curve, when orange peel flour concentration increased the oxidative rancidity decreased, in comparison of the higher values detected in the potato starch and carrageenan vertexes (Figure 2c).

Total polyphenols content in citrus peel and a consequent higher antioxidant effect, besides the higher dietetic fiber content, make citrus peels a potential ingredient to formulate functional foods (Rincón et al., 2005). In same manner, antioxidant activity of by-products obtained from industrial manipulation of citrus fruit has been widely demonstrated in cooked meat products (Viuda-Martos et al., 2009). Such activity is basically due to their composition mainly to phenolic compounds and flavonoids (Abd El-Khalek and Zahran, 2013; Escobedo-Avellaneda et al., 2013). The no presence of these types of compounds in carrageenan or potato starch resulted in higher rancidity values.

Texture Profile Analysis

For sausages hardness, linear terms of the model presented a highly significant ($p<0.01$) effect. In the regression equation (R^2= 99.74), potato starch had a stronger influence on this textural parameter, in comparison with orange peel flour or carrageenan (Table 3). This means that higher potato starch proportions resulted in harder sausages, where higher hardness values were perpendicular to the potato starch vertex (Figure 3a). Higher proportions of orange peel flour resulted in softer texture. In samples cohesiveness, linear terms had a highly significant ($p<0.01$) effect on texture, and the interaction orange peel flour with potato starch had a significantly ($p<0.05$) effect.

Table 3. Regression model and Analysis of Variance for the instrumental texture TPA of the different formulated sausages

Hardness (N)= 17.58 Orange peel +32.86 Starch +18.13 CGN, R^2= 99.74					
Source	DF	SS	MS	F	Pr>F
Orange peel	1	564,609	564,609	69.481	0.0001
Starch	1	1973.141	1973.141	242.810	0.0001
CGN	1	600.864	600.864	73.943	0.0001
Model	2	223.941	56.882	8.126	0.0037
Error	7	56.7652	8.1093		
Total	9	280.824			

Table 3. (Continued)

Cohesiveness= 0.3997 Orange peel +0.3740 Starch +0.3149 CGN +0.0149 Orange peel*Starch, R^2= 72.91					
Source	DF	SS	MS	F	Pr>F
Orange peel	1	0.2163	0.2163	187.268	0.0001
Starch	1	0.1895	0.1895	164,008	0.0001
CGN	1	0.1801	0.1801	155.877	0.0001
Orange peel*Starch	1	0.0001	0.0001	1.7002	0.0244
Model	3	0.0059	0.0019	21.1458	0.0653
Error	6	0.0069	0.0011		
Total	9	0.0128			
Resilience= 0.7158 Orange peel +0.7191 Starch +0.6657 CGN, R^2= 47.01					
Source	DF	SS	MS	F	Pr>F
Orange peel	1	0.9362	0.9362	1338.216	0.0001
Starch	1	0.9446	0.9446	1350.234	0.0001
CGN	1	0.8097	0.8097	1157.308	0.0001
Model	2	0.0026	0.0013	1.9090	0.2179
Error	7	0.0049	0.0007		
Total	9	0.0076			

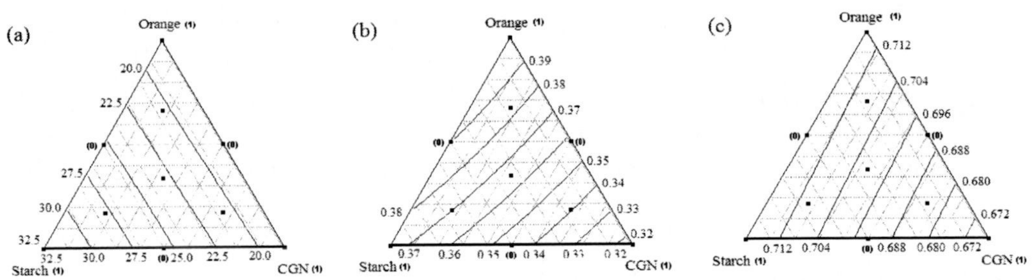

Figure 3. Isoresponse curve for: (a) hardness, (b) cohesiveness y (c) resilience in formulated sausages.

In the regression equation (R^2= 72.91) linear parameters had similar values, that in addition to the positive effect of the orange peel flour and potato starch interaction, increasing cohesiveness values (Table 3). In the isoresponse curves at higher orange peel flour proportions the sausages cohesiveness was higher, in comparison with carrageenan or potato starch (Figure 3b). In the resilience, linear terms had a highly significant effect ($p<0.01$) on this textural characteristic. In the regression equation (R^2= 74.01) the three components of the mixture had positive effect (Table 3). In the isoresponse curve at higher orange peel flour proportions the resilience values were higher (Figure 3c).

Although it has been reported that the fiber incorporation increased emulsified meat products hardness and cohesiveness (Fernández-Ginés et al., 2003; García et al., 2007; Petridis et al., 2013), at the employed experimental conditions, orange peel flour resulted in softer but more cohesive and resilient texture. On other hand, potato starch in emulsified meat products compensates the textural properties increasing protein matrix structure gel strength (Kerry et al., 1999, Aktaş and Gençcelep, 2006; Li and Yeh, 2002) resulting in this case in a harder, less cohesive and more resilient structure. Carrageenan incorporation increased hardness and cohesiveness of cooked sausages (Ayadi et al., 2009; Cierach et al., 2009). At the experimental conditions employed, pure carrageenan formulation obtained same hardness value than orange peel flour samples, but with lower cohesiveness and resilience values. Main differences between the studied extenders are their inherent diverse composition that determinate their functionality at sausages process conditions, like temperature and ionic strength.

For potato starch there are two main considerations. First, starch gelatinization is subject to differences between amylose and amylopectin biopolymers structure (as chains length, flexibility, regularity and tendency to self-aggregate), affecting solubility and thermodynamic compatibility (Tolstoguzov, 2003). Secondly, although potato starch is recommended in cooked meat products because swell easily due to their lower gelatinization and pasting temperatures (Murphy, 2000), salt presence modifies starch/meat complexes thermal properties (Defreitas et al., 1997; Li and Yeh, 2003). Salt repress starch granule swelling increasing gelatinization temperature (Bello-Pérez and Paredes-López, 1995). In this view, at cooked meat products environmental conditions starch gelatinization is affected since processing temperatures (70-72 °C) and salt content (2.0-2.5% = 0.5-0.6 M NaCl), potato starch granules are not able to completely gelatinize and swell, decreasing functionality and affecting in some degree cooked meat products water retention (García-García and Totosaus, 2008).

For carrageenans, water binding capacity, gel formation and thickening properties depend on their anionic character as result of the sulfate groups per repeating unit, where kappa carrageenan is employed in meat products for its gelling characteristics (Piculell, 2006). However, ionic composition of a food system is important for effective utilization of the carrageenan, where ions presence also has a dramatic effect on the hydration, setting or gelation and melting temperatures. As a carrageenan dispersion is heated, particles do not swell or hydrate until the temperature exceeds about 40–60 °C, but in meat brine sodium salt of kappa carrageenan will only fully hydrate at 55 °C, with a marked increase in viscosity followed by gelation below temperatures of 40-50 °C (Imeson, 2009). This implies that under meat processing conditions where meat products are of high ionic strength and/or reach internal temperatures of 65–70 °C, kappa-carrageenan may not be completely solubilized and may not achieve optimal gel network development on cooling (Shand et al., 1994). Since sodium is a non specific helix promoting cation for kappa-carrageenan (Imeson, 2009), the presence of other specific helix-promoting cations (potassium and/or calcium) improved kappa carrageenan functionality in low fat sodium reduced meat batters (Totosaus et al., 2004).

For fiber contained in peel flour, the structural components had a different influence by environmental conditions. Dietary fiber from fruits had better nutritional quality because, in hand, the content of bioactive compounds (antioxidants like flavonoids and carotenoids); and on the other hand, a higher overall fiber content (with a greater soluble/insoluble dietary fiber ratio), in comparison to fiber from cereals (Chou and Huang, 2003). Soluble components, as pectin and gums, are soluble dietary fiber; and insoluble materials as cellulose, hemicelluloses and lignin are non soluble dietary fiber (Thebaudin et al., 1997). Key property of fruit fiber (cell wall matrix as principal structural component) is hydration that summarizes the ability to swell, bind water, enhance viscosity and prevent syneresis (Fischer, 2003). The swelling capacity of fiber was not influenced by salt presence (1 M) because cell wall structures differences (different hydration properties). Cellulose cell walls are rigid and hydrophobic, whereas parenchymatous cell walls are rich in hydrophilic pectin and highly hydrated *in vivo*. In cellulose cell walls the main factor associated to hydration is probably the solvation of its constituent polysaccharides, counteracted by the lignin/cellulose network. In parenchymal structures, electrostatic forces of the constituent pectin are prevalent, solvating charged ionogenic groups provoking an electrostatic repulsion between adjacent carboxyl groups (Renard et al., 1994). In this view, is expected that orange peel flour, rich in fiber, was not affected by emulsified meat products processing conditions, as temperature or ion strength, having a better functional performance retaining water and improving texture.

Conclusion

Most employed meat extenders like potato starch or kappa-carrageenan do not had the optimum performance at the emulsified meatprocess conditions, like temperature and salt concentration. The fiber content (around 38%) in orange peel flour presented a better performance at the experimental conditions employed, as compared to potato starch or carrageenan, and was not influenced by either temperature or salt concentration as emulsified meat process conditions. Orange peel flour increased moisture and retained more water (as total moisture and liberated water) than potato starch or carrageenan, besides decrease the oxidative rancidity in cooked sausages. Minimal changes in color were observed by replace potato starch and/or carrageenan by orange peel flour. Orange peel can replace potato starch at lower amount to reach close hardness values. Softer and less compact samples (lower cohesiveness and resilience) were obtained with carrageenan, as compared to orange peel flour. Theseresults means that orange peel flour as a cheap and viable fiber source can replace more expensive meat extenders, as potato starch or carrageenan.

Acknowledgments

This work was supported into the project “Aprovechamiento de subproductos agroindustriales como fuente de fibra y su posible utilización como prebióticos en productos cárnicos”, PICSO 11-21 ICyTDF, México City, México.

References

Abd El-Khalek, H.H. and Zahran, D.A.2013. Utilization of fruit by-product in ground meat preservation. *Food Sci. Qual. Manage.*,11: 49-60.

Aktaş N. and Gençcelep, H. 2006 Effect of starch type and its modifications on physicochemical properties of bologna-type sausage produced with sheep tail fat. *Meat Sci.*,74: 404-408.

[AOAC]Official Methods of Analysis of AOAC International.16th edition. Gaithersburg, AOAC International. (1999)

Ayadi, M.A., Kechaou, A., Makni, I. and Attia, H. 2009. Influence of carrageenan addition on turkey meat sausages properties. *J. Food Eng.*,93: 278-283.

Balasundram, N., Sundram, K. and Samman, S. 2006. Phenolic compounds in plants and agri-industrial by-products: antioxidant activity, occurrence, and potential uses. *Food Chem.*, 99: 191-203.

Bello-Pérez, L.A. and Paredes-López, O.1995. Starch and amylopectin: Effect of solutes on their calorimetric behavior. *Food Chem.*,53: 243-247.

Bourne, M.C. 1978. Texture profile analysis. *Food Technol.*,32(4): 62-66, 72.

Chou, C.F. and Huang, Y.L. 2003. Comparison of the chemical composition and physical properties of different fiber prepared from the peel of *Citrus sinensis* L. Cv. Liucheng. *J. Agric. Food. Chem.*, 51: 2615-2618.

Cierach, M., Modzelewska-Kapituła, M. and Szaciło, K. 2009. The influence of carrageenan on the properties of low-fat frankfurters. *Meat Sci.*,82: 295-299.

Cornell, J.A. 1980. Experiments with Mixtures: Design Models, and the Analysis of Mixture Data. John Wiley & Sons, New York, pp. 2-63.

Defreitas, Z. Sebranek, J.G., Olson, D.G. and Carr, J.M. 1997. Carrageenan effects on thermal stability of meat proteins. *J. Food Sci.*,62: 539-543.

Dzieszuk, W., Dworecka, E. and Szmańko, T. 2005. The effect of added modified starch on quality of comminuted scalded sausages. *Acta Sci. Pol., Technol. Aliment.*,4: 111-121.

Escobedo-Avellaneda, Z., Gutiérrez-Uribe, J., Valdez-Fragoso, A., Torres, J.A. and Welti-Chanes, J. 2014. Phytochemicals and antioxidant activity of juice, flavedo, albedo and comminuted orange.*J. Functional Foods,* 6: 470-481.

Fernández-Ginés, J.M., Fernández-López, J., Sayas-Barberá, E., Sendra, E., and Pérez-Álvarez, J.A. 2003. Effect of storage conditions on quality characteristics of bologna sausages made with citrus fiber. *J. Food Sci.*,68: 710-715.

Fischer, J. 2009. Fruit fibers in Fiber Ingredients. Food Applications and Health Benefits, ed. Cho SS, and Samuel P. CRC Press, Boca Raton, pp. 427-438.

García, M.L., Cáceres, E. and Selgas, M.D. 2007. Utilisation of fruit fibres in conventional and reduced-fat cooked-meat sausages. *J. Sci. Food Agric.*,87: 624-631.

García-García, E. and Totosaus, A. 2008. Low-fat sodium-reduced sausages: Effect of the interaction between locust bean gum, potato starch and κ-carrageenan by a mixture design approach. *Meat Sci.*,78: 406-413.

Imeson, A.P. 2009. Carrageenan and furcellan in Handbook of Food Hydrocolloids, 2nd edition, ed. Phillips GO, and Williams PA. Woodhead Publishing, Cambridge, pp. 164-185.

Jauregui, C.A., Regenstein, J.M. and Baker, R.C. 1981. A simple centrifugal method for measuring expressible moisture, a water-binding property of muscle foods. *J. Food Sci.*,46: 1271-1273.

Kerry, J.F. and Kerry, J.P. 2006. Producing low-fat meat products in Improving the Fat Content of Foods, ed. Williams C, and Buttriss J. Woodhead Publishing, Cambridge, pp. 336-379.

Kerry, J.F., Morrissey, P.A. and Buckley, D.J.1999. The rheological properties of exudates from cured porcine muscle: effects of added polysaccharides and whey protein/polysaccharide blends. *J. Sci. Food Agric.*,79: 1260-1266.

Lario, Y., Sendra, E., García-Pérez, J., Fuentes, C., Sayas-Barberá, E., Fernández-López, J. and Pérez-Álvarez, J.A.2004. Preparation of high dietary fiber powder from lemon juice by-products. *Inn. Food Sci. Emerg. Technol.*, 5: 113-117.

Lawlor, J.B., Sheehy, P.J.A., Kerry, J.P., Buckley, D.J. and Morrissey, P.A. 2000. Measuring oxidative stability of beef muscles obtained from animals supplemented with vitamin E using conventional and derivative spectrophotometry. *J. Food Sci.*,65: 1138-1141.

Li, J.-Y. and Yeh, A.-I.2003. Effects of starch properties on rheological characteristics of starch/meat complexes. *J. Food Eng.*,57: 287-294.

Li, J.-Y. and Yeh, A.-I.2002. Functions of starch in formation of starch/meat composite during heating. *J. Texture Stud.*,33: 341-366.

Liu, H., Xiong, Y.L., Jiang, L. and Kong, B.2008. Fat reduction in emulsion sausage using an enzyme-modified potato starch.*J. Sci. Food Agric.*,88: 1632-1637.

Mehta, N., Ahlawat, S.S., Sharma, D.P. and Dabur, R.S.2013. Novel trends in development of dietary fiber rich meat products–a critical review. *J. Food Sci. Technol.* DOI: 10.1007/s13197-013-1010-2.

Moraes-Crizel, T., Jablonski, A., Oliveira-Rios, A., Rech, R. and Hickmann-Flôres, R.2013. Dietary fiber from orange byproducts as a potential fat replacer. *LWT-Food Sci. Technol.*,53: 9-14.

Murphy, P. 2000. Starch in Handbook of Food Hydrocolloids, ed. Phillips GO, and Williams PA. Woodhead Publishing, Cambridge, pp. 41-65.

Petridis, D., Raizi, P. and Ritzoulis, C. 2013. Influence of citrus fiber, rice bran and collagen on the texture and organoleptic properties of low-fat frankfurters. *J. Food Proc Pres.*,38: 1759-1771.

Piculell, L. 2006. Gelling carrageenans in Food Polysaccharides and Their Applications, 2nd edition, ed. Stephen AM, Phillips GO, and Williams PA. CRC Press, Boca Raton, pp. 239-287.

Renard, C.M.G.C., Crépeau, M.-J. and Thibault, J.-F. 1994. Influence of ionic strength, pH and dielectric constant on hydration properties of native and modified fibres from sugar-beet and wheat bran. *Ind. Crops Prod.*,3: 75-84.

Rincón, A.M., Vásquez, A., Padilla, M. and Fanny, C. 2005. Composicionquimica y compuestos bioactivos de las harinas de cascaras de naranja (*Citrus sinensis*), mandarina (*Citrus reticulata*) y toronja (*Citrus paradisi*) cultivadas en Venezuela. *Arch. Latinoam. Nutr.*, 55: 305-310 (2005).

Shand, P.J., Sofos, J.N. and Schmidt, G.R.1994. Differential scanning calorimetry of beef/kappa-carrageenan mixtures. *J. FoodSci.*, 59: 711-715.

[SIAP] 2013. Sistema de Información Agroalimentaria y Pesquera, Atlas Agroalimentario. Secretaria de Agricultura, Ganadería, Desarrollo Rural, Pesca y Alimentación, SAGARPA, México. http://www.siap.gob.mx/atlas2013/index.html.

Szczceniak, A.S.1963. Classification of textural characteristics.*J. Food Sci.*,28: 385-389.

Thebaudin, J.Y., Levebvre, A.C., Harrington, M. and Bourgeois, C.M.1997.Dietary fibers: nutritional and technological interests. *Trends Food Sci. Technol.*,8: 41-48.

Tolstoguzov, V.2003.Thermodynamic considerations of starch functionality in foods. *CarbohPolym.*, 51: 99-111.

Totosaus, A., Alfaro-Rodríguez, R.H. and Pérez-Chabela, M.L. 2004. Fat and sodium chloride reduction in sausages using κ-carrageenan and other salts. *Int. J. Food Sci. Nutrit.*, 55: 371-380.

Trius, A., Sebranek, J.G. and Lanier, T.1996. Carrageenans and their use in meat products. *Crit. Rev. Food Sci. Nutrit.*, 36: 69-85.

Verma, A.K. and Banerjee, R. 2010. Dietary fibre as functional ingredient in meat products: a novel approach for healthy living –A review. *J. Food Sci. Technol.*,47: 247-257.

Viuda-Martos, M., Fernández-López, J., Sayas-Barberá, E., Sendra, E., Navarro, C. and Pérez-Álvarez, J.A.2009. Citrus co-products as technological strategy to reduce residual nitrite content in meat products. *J. Food Sci.*,74: 93-100.

Yalinkiliç, B., Kaban, G. and Kaya, M. 2012. The effects of different levels of orange fiber and fat on microbiological, physical, chemical and sensorial properties of sucuk. *Food Microbiol.*,29: 255-259.

Zhang, L. and Barbut, S.2005. Effects of regular and modified starches on cooked pale, soft, and exudative; normal; and dry, firm, and dark breast meat batters. *Poultry Sci.*,84: 789-796.

Zipser, M.W. and Watts, B.M.1962. A modified 2-thiobarbituric acid (TBA) method for the determination of malonaldehyde in cured meats. *Food Technol.*, 16(7): 102-104.

In: Dietary Fiber
Editor: Marvin E. Clemens

ISBN: 978-1-63463-655-1
© 2015 Nova Science Publishers, Inc.

Chapter 10

MICROBIAL EXOPOLYSACCHARIDES AS ALTERNATIVE SOURCES OF DIETARY FIBERS WITH INTERESTING FUNCTIONAL AND HEALTHY PROPERTIES

Habib Chouchane[1,*], Mohamed Neifar[2,†], Noura Raddadi[3], Fabio Fava[3], Ahmed Slaheddine Masmoudi[1] and Ameur Cherif[1]

[1]Laboratory of Biotechnology and Bio-Geo Resources Valorization, Higher Institute for Biotechnology, Biotechpole Sidi Thabet, University of Manouba, Ariana, Tunisia
[2]Laboratory of Microorganisms and Active Biomolecules, Faculty of Sciences of Tunis, University of Tunis El Manar, Tunis, Tunisia
[3]Department of Civil, Chemical, Environmental and Materials Engineering (DICAM), Alma Mater Studiorum-University of Bologna, Italy

ABSTRACT

Traditional polysaccharides obtained from plants may suffer from a lack of reproducibility in their rheological properties, purity, supply and cost. Most of the used plant polysaccharides are chemically modified to improve their characteristics. Microbial exopolysaccharides (EPSs) are principally composed of carbohydrate polymers, and they are produced by many microorganisms including bacteria, yeasts and fungi. Microorganisms can synthesize EPSs and excrete them out of cell either as soluble or insoluble polymers. These EPSs are able not only to protect the microorganisms themselves against desiccation, phage attack, antibiotics or toxic compounds, but also can be applied in several biotechnological applications. In food products they increase the dietary fiber content and can be used as viscosifiers, stabilizers, emulsifiers or gelling agents to improve physical and structural properties of water and oil holding capacity,

* Habib Chouchane: Laboratory of Biotechnology and Bio-Geo Resources Valorization, Higher Institute for Biotechnology, Biotechpole Sidi Thabet, University of Manouba, 2020 Ariana, Tunisia. Phone: 00216 70527882 / 71537040, fax: 00216 70527882 / 71537044, e-mail: chouchane_habib@voila.fr.
† Mohamed Neifar: Laboratory of Microorganisms and Active Biomolecules, Faculty of Sciences of Tunis, University of Tunis El Manar, 2092 Tunis, Tunisia. E-mail: Mohamed_naifar@yahoo.com.

viscosity, texture, sensory characteristics and shelf-life. EPSs are used as additives in various foods, such as dairy products, jams and jellies, wine and beer, fishery and meat products, icings and glazes, frozen foods and bakery products. Over the past few decades, interest in using microbial EPSs in food processing has been increasing because of main reasons such as easy production, better rheological and stability characteristics, cost effectiveness and supply. Dextran, xanthan, pullulan, curdlan, levan, gellan and alginate are the main examples of industrially important microbial exopolysaccharides. They also play crucial role in conferring beneficial physiological effects on human health, such as the ability to lower pressure and to reduce lipid level in blood. Furthermore, these EPSs exhibit antitumor, immunomodulating, antioxidant and antibacterial properties. The utility of various biopolymers are dependent on their monosaccharide composition, type of linkages present, degree of branching and molecular weight. In the present chapter, an attempt was taken to recapitulate the most important polysaccharides isolated from microorganisms as well as the main methods for microbial exopolysaccharide production, purification and structural characterization. In addition, the functional and healthy benefits of EPSs and their applications in food industry were discussed.

Keywords: Microbial exopolysaccharides, dietary fibers, human health, functional properties, food applications

INTRODUCTION

Microbial exopolysaccharides (EPSs) have been recognized as high value biomacromolecules for the last two decades. EPSs of microbial origin might represent a valid alternative to the currently used plant gums considering that their properties are almost identical. In other cases, the microbial EPSs have unusual molecular structures and peculiar conformations, thus conferring unique interesting health and functional properties with potential use in food industry (figure 1) (De Oliveira et al., 2007; Shih et al., 2009; Annarita et al., 2011; Nwodo et al., 2012).

EPSs have been isolated from different genera of bacteria, archaea, fungi and algae mainly belonging to mesophilic, thermophilic and halophilic groups (Kalogiannis et al., 2003; Ravella et al., 2010; Tapan, 2012). The physiological role of these molecules are not yet clearly understood, although it is generally recognized that EPSs are not normally used as energy and carbon sources by the producing microorganism. They can serve for a variety of functions including cell recognition and interaction, adherence to solid surfaces, survival to adverse conditions and biofilm formation. In some cases, EPS enables the bacteria to capture nutrients (Ruas-Madiedo et al., 2002; Lin et al., 2011).

EPSs biosynthesis and accumulation generally take place after the growth phase of the microorganism in response to limitation of nutrients such as nitrogen and phosphate (Annarita et al., 2011). EPSs biosynthesis can be divided into three main steps: the assimilation of a carbon substrate, intracellular synthesis of the polysaccharides and EPS exudation out of the cell. EPSs are divided into two classes, homo- and hetero-EPSs. Homo-EPSs are composed of one type of monosaccharide repeating unit (e.g., pullulan, levan, curdlan, cellulose, dextran) while heteropolysaccharides are composed of two or more types of monosaccharides (e.g., gellan, xanthan, alginate, chitosan) (Patel and Prajapati, 2013; Madhuri and Prabhakar 2014).

Microbial EPS production mainly depends on the type of microbial strain used, physical conditions maintained during fermentation and on kind of media components (Yang and He

2008; Donot et al., 2012). EPS production is generally favoured by high carbon and low nitrogen substrate ratio (Lim et al., 2004; Luo et al., 2009). Approaches for the reduction of production costs might involve using cheaper substrates, improving product yield by optimizing fermentation conditions, or developing higher yielding strains (Donot et al., 2012; Mahapatra and Banerjee, 2013). Microbial EPS production offers benefits such as the production in a matter of days compared to many months in the case of plants, the possibility of utilising industrial wastes as carbon and nitrogen substrates and the absence of competition with arable land.

The revised definition of dietary fibers not only includes nondigestible plant polysaccharides, but also their analogues, such as microbial EPSs (Chung, 2000; Martensson et al., 2003). Foods containing EPS fibers are known for their ability to prevent or relieve constipation. But also, they can provide other health benefits such as helping to maintain a healthy weight and lowering risk of coronary heart disease, diabetes, obesity, and some forms of cancer (Mann and Cummings, 2009; Luo et al., 2009; Ramberg et al., 2010; Lin, et al., 2011; He et al., 2012).

When added to food (bakery fillings, confections, dairy products, dessert gels, icings and glazes, jams and jellies, low-fat spreads, sauces and structured foods), microbial EPSs show functions as thickeners, stabilizers, emulsifiers, gelling agents, and water binding agents (Freitas, et al., 2011; Nwodo et al., 2012; Patel and Prajapati, 2013; Tabibloghmany and Ehsandoost, 2014).

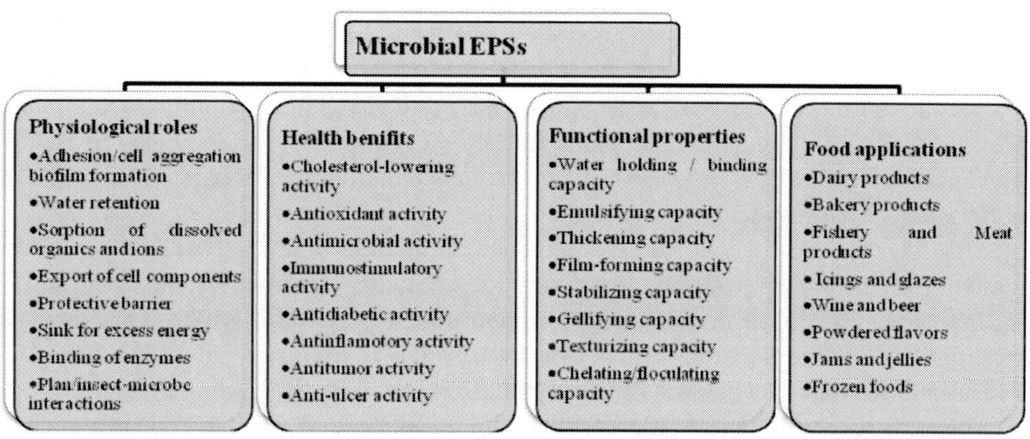

(De Oliveira et al., 2007; Rehm, 2009; Shih et al., 2009; Annarita et al., 2011; Elizaquivel, et al., 2011; Freitas et al., 2011; Poli et al., 2011; Nwodo et al., 2012; Patel and Prajapati, 2013; Tabibloghmany and Ehsandoost, 2014).

Figure 1. An overview of the physiological roles, health benefits, functional properties and food applications of microbial EPSs.

The functional properties of EPSs including viscosity rely on their molecular mass, monosaccharide composition, primary structure and interaction with food components, principally proteins. They also contribute to conservation, and improve the appearance, stability and rheological properties of novel food products (Patel and Prajapati, 2013).

The importance that EPSs has gained in food industries argue the development of other strategies to improve the total amount produced. Some of these strategies are their *in situ* production in food matrices and their *in vitro* production by the use of immobilized enzymes (Werning et al., 2012).

This chapter provides a brief summary of the current knowledge pertaining to the microbial EPSs, from sources biosynthesis to food applications, detailing their sources, structures, production processes, functional properties and human health benefits.

I. Sources and Physiological Roles of Microbial Exopolysaccharides

Many bacteria (Gram-positive and Gram-negative bacteria) and cyanobacteria, yeasts, fungi and algal cells are able to synthesize and excrete EPSs. Commercially, the most important EPSs are from bacterial and fungal origin (table 1). Three bacterial species were identified as strong producers of EPSs with production yields above or equal to 70 g/l. These bacteria are *Agrobacterium sp.* and *Alcaligenes faecalis* producing 76 and 72 g/l of curdlan, respectively (Wu et al., 2008; Shih et al., 2009) and *Bacillus subtilus* natto producing 70.6 g/l of levan (Shih et al., 2010). EPS-producing microorganisms have been isolated from different natural aquatic and terrestrial sources. Effluents from the sugar, paper or food industries as well as wastewater plants characterised with high carbon/nitrogen ratio are also known to contain microorganisms producing EPSs (Singha, 2012). Extremophilic microorganisms isolated from deep-sea hydrothermal vents, Antarctic ecosystems, saline lakes and geothermal springs have been recently investigated as potential sources of precious EPSs (table 2). Thermophilic bacteria as *Geobacillus tepidamans* V264 are able to produce high molecular weights and thermostable EPSs, some of them start to degrade at about 280°C (Kambourova et al., 2009). The most common halophilic EPS producers are bacteria belonging to the genus *Halomonas*, particularly, *H. alkaliantarctica, H. stenophila* (Amjres et al., 2015), *H. ventosae* and *H. anticariensis* (Mata et al., 2006).

EPSs synthesized by *Halomonas* strains had an unusual high sulphate level and a large amount of uronic acids responsible for their good gelifying properties (Nicolaus et al., 2010; Annarita et al., 2011). The greatly variable composition, structure, biosynthesis and functional properties of EPSs from extremophiles have been widely investigated but only a few of them have been industrially developed (Annarita et al., 2011).

The precise physiological role of microbial EPSs depends on the producer niche. In general, microorganisms produce EPSs as a strategy for growing, adhering to solid surfaces, and surviving adverse conditions (Nwodo et al., 2012). The ability of a microorganism to surround itself with a highly hydrated EPS layer may provide it with protection against harsh condition such as desiccation, osmotic stress, antibiotics, toxic compounds or against possible predation by protozoans, phagocytosis and phage attack (Kumar, et al., 2007; Ganzle and Schwab, 2009; Nwodo et al., 2012).

Table 1. Important microbial EPSs and their major sources

Microorganisms	EPSs	EPS concentrations (g L−1)	References
Bacteria			
Agrobacterium sp.	Curdlan	76	Shih et al., 2009
Alcaligenes faecalis	Curdlan	72	Wu et al., 2008
Bacillus subtilis natto	Levan	70.6	Shih et al., 2010
Leuconostoc mesenteroides	Dextran	54-55	Vedyashkina et al., 2005
Xanthomonas campestris	Xanthan	53	Kalogiannis et al., 2003
Zymonas mobilis	Levan	50	De Oliveira et al., 2007
Agrobacterium tumefaciens	Succinoglycan	42	Stredansky and Conti, 1999
Sphingomonas paucimobilis	Gellan	35.7	Nampoothiri et al., 2003
Acetobacter xylinum	Cellulose	15	Hwang et al., 1999
Azobacter vinelandii	Alginate	9.5	Mejía et al., 2010
Streptococcus sp.	Hyaluronan	6-7	Boeriu et al., 2013
Yeasts and fungi			
Aureobasidium pullulans	Pullulan	52.5	Ravella et al., 2010
Sclerotium rolfsii	Scleroglucan	23.8	Survase et al., 2007
Schizophyllum commune	Schizophyllan	8.0	Kumari et al., 2008
Rhodotorula acheniorum	Mannan	6.2	Pavlova et al., 2005
Sporobolomyces sp.	Galactan	5.6	Pavlova et al., 2004
Gongronella butleri	Chitosan	1.2	Streit et al., 2009

EPSs are also crucial in the aggregate formation, in the mechanism of adhesion to surfaces, in the uptake of nutrients, in cryoprotection, in plant-microbe and insect-microbe interactions, etc. (Figure 1).

The EPSs biosynthesis is a process that requires a noticeable energy cost of up to 70% of total energy reserve, representing a significant carbon investment for microorganisms. But, the benefits related to EPSs biosynthesis are higher than costs considering the increasing growth and survival of microorganisms in their presence (Poli et al., 2011).

II. Composition and Structural Features of Microbial Exopolysaccharides

Polysaccharides show considerable diversity in their composition and structure. They are generally classified as homo- and hetero-EPSs based on their monomeric composition. Table 3 summarizes the chemical characteristics of major bacterial and fungal EPSs. Homo-EPSs are composed of one type of monosaccharide repeating unit as D-glucopyranose (glucans) and D-fructopyranose (fructans) (Werning et al., 2012; Tabibloghmany and Ehsandoost, 2014).

These polysaccharides usually show high molecular masses (up to 107 KDa), and have various degrees and kinds of branching, linking sites and chain length.

Table 2. Examples of characterized exopolysaccharides from extremophilic microorganisms

Microorganisms	Extreme environment source	Description of EPS	References
Halomonas sp.	Soil samples from Çamaltı Saltern area in Turkey	Levan polymer (the repeating unit was composed of β-(2,6)-D-fructofuranosyl residues)	Poli et al., 2009
H. anticariensis	Saline soils	Glucose Mannose Galacturonic acid	Mata et al., 2006
H. ventosae and *H. anticariensis*	Saline soils in Jaén, southeastern Spain	Glucose galactose mannose as main components	Mata et al., 2006
H. stenophila	Saline-wetland in Brikcha, Morocco	A sulphated heteropolysaccharide composed of glucose glucuronic acid, mannose, fucose, galactose and rhamnose	Amjres et al., 2015
H. alkaliantarctica	Salt lake in Cape Russell in Antarctica	Glc:Fru:GlcN:GalN (1.0:0.7:0.3:trace)	Poli et al., 2004; Poli et al., 2007
Pseudomonas sp.	Marine sediment, Antarctica	Glucose galactose and fucose	Carrion et al., 2014
Alteromonas macleodii	Water sample from Arabian sea	High EPS yield (23.4 g/1) when 15% lactose was used as substrate	Mehta et al., 2014
Haloferax mediterranei	Mediterranean Sea	A high molecular weight sulfated polysaccharide	Parolis et al., 1996
Geobacillus sp.	Sediment in marine hot spring near the seashore of Maronti, Ischia Island, Italy	A pentasaccharide repeating unit (two of them with a gluco-galacto configuration and three with a manno configuration.	Nicolaus et al., 2002
Bacillus thermodenitrificans	Shallow hydrothermal vent, Vulcano Island, Italy	Trisaccharide repeating unit and a manno-pyranosidic configuration. Man:Glc (1:0.2)	Arena et al., 2009
Bacillus licheniformis	Shallow marine hot spring, Vulcano Island, Italy	Man is the main monosaccharide. Tetrasaccharide repeating unit and a manno-pyranosidic configuration	Arena et al., 2006
Thermococcus litoralis	Shallow submarine thermal spring	Man is the only monosaccharide	Rinker and Kelly, 2000
Thermus aquaticus	Biofilm	Tetrasaccharide- repeating units of galactofuranose, galactopyranose, and N-acetylgalactosamine (1:1:2) and lacked acidic sugars.	Lin et al., 2011
Pseudoalteromonas sp.	Deep-sea hydrothermal vent	Sulfated heteropolysaccharide, high in uronic acids, with pyruvate and acetate	Colliec-Joult et al., 2004
	Southern Ocean	Sulfated heteropolysaccharide, high in uronic acids with acetyl and succinyl groups	Mancuso-Nichols et al., 2004
	Antarctica	Sulfated heteropolysaccharide, high in uronic acids with acetyl groups	Mancuso-Nichols et al., 2004

Table 3. Basic characteristics of the most important microbial exopolysaccharides

EPS	Monomers	Charge	Types of Glycosidic linkages*
Xanthan	Glucose Mannose Glucuronic acid	Anionic	β-1,4; (β-1,2; α-1,3)
Gellan	Glucose Rhamnose Glucuronic acid	Anionic	β-1,4; α-1,4; β-1,3
Alginate	Guluronic acid Mannuronic acid	Anionic	β-1,4
Succinoglycan	Galactose Glucose	Acidic	β-1,3; β-1,4- β-1,6
Hyaluronan	Glucuronic acid Acetylglucosamine	Anionic	β-1,4; β-1,3
Chitosan	Glucosamine Acetyl-glucosamine	Anionic	β-1,4
Chitin	Acetyl-glucosamine	Anionic	β-1,4
Reuteran	Glucose	Neutral	α-1,4
Cellulose	Glucose	Neutral	β-1,4
Curdlan	Glucose	Neutral	β-1,3
Dextran	Glucose	Neutral	α-1,6; (α-1,3; α-1,4; α-1,2)
Mutan	Glucose	Neutral	α-1,3
Alternan	Glucose	Neutral	α-1, 6; α-1, 3; (α-1, 3)
Pullulan	Glucose	Neutral	α-1,4; α-1,6
Scleroglucan	Glucose	Neutral	β-1,3; (β-1,6)
Schizophyllan	Glucose	Neutral	β-1,3; β-1,6
Levan	Fructose	Neutral	β-2,6; (β-1,2)
Inulin	Fructose	Neutral	β-1,2; (β-2,6)
Galactan	galactopyranose	Neutral	α-1,3
Mannan	Mannose	Neutral	α-1,2; α-1,3/α-1,6 (α-1,2; α-1,3)

*In parenthesis are linkages that are present in lesser degree, and/or in side chains.
Smelcerovic et al., 2008; Freitas et al., 2011; Donot et al., 2012; Nwodo et al. 2012.

According to their structure, the fructans are divided into two groups: inulins (linked β-2,1) and levans (linked β-2,6). Glucans are classified into α- and β-D-glucans. Taking in to account of the linkages in the main chain, the α-glucans are subdivided into reuterans (α-1,4), dextrans (α-1,6), mutans (α-1,3), alternans (α-1,3 and α-1,6) and pullulan (α-1,4; α-1,6). β-D-glucans include cellulose (β-1,3) and curdlan (β-1,3) that have been approved as a food additive by the Food and Drug Administration (Mcintosh et al., 2005). Hetero- EPSs contain two or more types of monosaccharides and are often present as multiple copies of oligosaccharides with three to eight residues (xanthan, gellan, alginate, hyaluronan). Hetero-EPSs are linear or branched, with variable molecular masses (up to 106 KDa). The monosaccharides are present as the α- or β-anomer in the pyranose or furanose form and D-glucose, D-galactose and L-rhamnose are the most commonly encountered.

In few cases, N-acetylglucosamine, manose, fucose, glucuronic acid and noncarbohydrate substituents (phosphate, acetyl and glycerol) are involved in the composition (Mozzi et al., 2006; Werning et al., 2012; Mahapatra and Banerjee, 2013; Patel and Prajapati, 2013).

Studies on microbial EPS structure are crucial not only for understanding their physico-chemical and biological properties, but also for the optimal exploitation in several industrial applications.

III. Biosynthesis of Microbial Exopolysaccharides

Microbial EPS biosynthesis is a multi-step process and needs enzymes involved in, (i) the formation of nucleotide sugar precursors which are the donors of sugars to the repeat unit, (ii) glycosyltransferases catalyzing the sequential transfer of sugars for the repeating unit formation, (iii) proteins implicated in the export of these oligosaccharide units from the cytoplasmic to the periplasmic face of the microbial membrane and (iv) enzymes involved in EPS polymerization and secretion to the extracellular medium. Other enzymes taking part in EPS acetylation and/or other modifications, and regulatory genes to control EPS production are also required (Czaczyk and Myszka, 2007; Tsuda, 2013; Patel and Prajapati, 2013; Tabibloghmany and Ehsandoost., 2014). As reported by Freitas et al. (2011), EPSs biosynthesis can be controlled at three different levels: synthesis of sugar nucleotide precursors; assembly of the repeating unit; and polymerization and export. The change of the expression of single genes or groups of genes can be used to increase the conversion efficiency of the chemical entities involved, and therefore, enhance EPS yields. More understanding of the molecular organization and of the factors regulating expression of EPS will make possible promoting EPS production and to increase the number of possibilities for modifying their structure and function. For a small number of homopolysaccharides, including dextrans and levans, the biosynthesis process is extracellular and needs the specific substrate sucrose. Highly specific glycosyl transferases (e.g., dextran sucrase and levan sucrase, respectively) are involved in the polymerization reaction (Tsuda, 2013; Tabibloghmany and Ehsandoost, 2014). The polymerization energy comes from the hydrolysis of sucrose. The polysaccharide can be produced either using whole bacterial cell cultures or immobilized enzyme preparations (De Vuyst and Degeest, 1999).

IV. Production of Microbial Exopolysaccharides

Microbial EPS production mainly depends on the type of microbial strain used, physical conditions maintained during fermentation, and type of medium components (figure 2). Production of most microbial EPSs use submerged culture techniques in Erlenmeyer flasks or in stirred tank fermentors. Many researchers used statistical methods including screening designs (e.g., fractional factorial design, Plackett-Burman design) and response surface methodology (e.g., Box-Behnken design, central composite design) for optimization of microbial EPS production (Donot et al., 2012; Liu et al., 2011; Zhang, 2011; Mahapatra and Banerjee, 2013; Qiang et al., 2013; Finore et al., 2014). EPS production could be maximized either at its late exponential stage or its early stationary stage of growth.

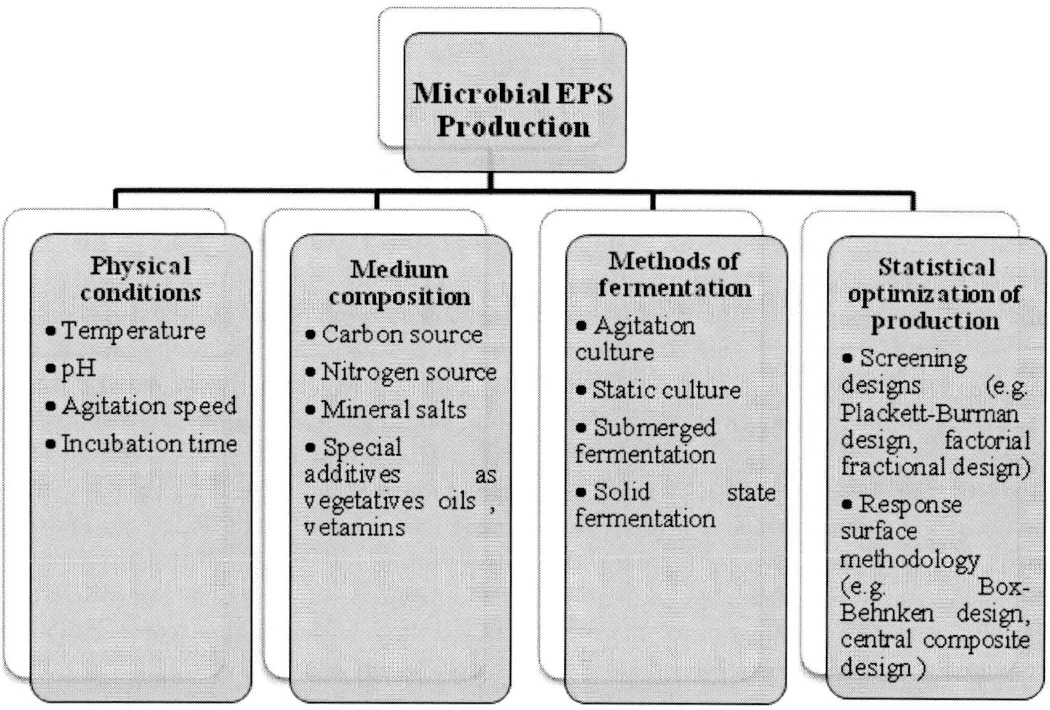

Donot et al., 2012; Mahapatra and Banerjee, 2013.

Figure 2. A schematic illustration of the main factors on which microbial exopolysaccharide production depends and some statistical approaches used to optimize their levels.

The production intensity of microbial EPSs is highly dependant on the nitrogen and carbon sources used and their concentration. In the majority of studies glucose and sucrose have been selected as the most suitable carbon sources for the production of microbial EPSs. The concentration of selected carbon source in the culture media is also a crucial factor for this production. Many findings indicate that, carbon source concentration between 20 to 60 g/L was suggested to enhance microbial EPSs production (Elisashvili et al., 2009; Mahapatra and Banerjee, 2013) but some exceptions were also reported (Xu et al., 2003; Tavares et al., 2005). Combined carbon sources can induce microbial EPSs production as demonstrated by Zhang et al. (2002). Nitrogen supplementation is another factor that is reported to induce EPS production. Both inorganic and organic nitrogen sources were tested in several studies to find the suitable one. Among the organic sources, peptone and yeast extract were tested mostly. Concerning the inorganic sources, ammonium chloride and ammonium sulphate are commonly studied. Many findings indicate that in the presence of organic nitrogen sources, microorganisms produce more EPSs in comparison to inorganic nitrogen supplements. Excluding a few studies, researchers found that in comparison to carbon sources, low nitrogen level is needed by microorganisms for EPS production and concentrations between 1-10 g/L are often sufficient (Mahapatra and Banerjee, 2013). Effects of phosphate source, some minerals and other additives including vegetable oils, fatty acids, surfactants, and vitamins on EPS production were also studied and reported (Yang and He, 2008; Zhang and Cheung, 2011).

V. Recovery, Purification and Characterization of Microbial EPS

The critical steps involved in the recovery, purification and structural characterization of microbial EPS are shown in Figure 3. EPS purification from microbial culture means elimination of producer microorganisms and their secreted metabolites as well as components of the growth media (Freitas et al., 2011; Donot et al., 2012; Patel and Prajapati, 2013). The first step of purification of EPS depends on the microbial growth medium used for its production. In complex media, the first requirement is the elimination of proteins. For their removal, precipitation with trichloroacetic acid (TCA) as well as treatment with proteases are the most commonly used methods. After that, the supernatant is usually subjected to one or more cycles of precipitation with ethanol, methanol, isopropanol or acetone and then dialysed to remove the low molecular weight contaminants. After lyophilisation of the samples, the EPS is further purified using chromatographic techniques (Size-exclusion chromatography; ion-exchange chromatography) (Freitas et al., 2011; Donot et al., 2012; Patel and Prajapati, 2013). The apparent average molecular weight can be estimated after size-exclusion chromatography fractionation. A calibration curve is performed by fractionation of standards and used for the determination of the molecular weight. The monomeric composition and structure of microbial EPSs were usually evaluated by different experimental analysis of intact EPSs, hydrolyzed or partially hydrolyzed EPSs, or their derivatives.

In general, these studies are analyzed through Fourier Transform Infrared spectroscopy (FTIR), paper chromatography, *high performance* liquid *chromatography* (HPLC), gas-liquid chromatography (GLC), gas-liquid chromatography-mass spectrometry (GLC-MS), Nuclear magnetic resonance spectrometry (NMR) and atomic force microscopy (AFM).

VI. Healthy and Functional Properties of Microbial EPSs

Various microbial EPSs, including alginate, pectins, gellan gum, xanthan gum and chitosan can function as dietary fibers and they would be expected to reduce intestinal absorption and cardiovascular disease risk, modulate colonic microflora and elevate colonic barrier function (Soh et al., 2003; Tok and Aslim, 2010; Patel and Prajapati, 2013). From a physiological standpoint, the main function of a dietary fiber is to lower cholesterol levels and to promote the loss of body weight through a reduction of intestinal lipid absorption (Tok and Aslim, 2010; Tsuda, 2013). The microbial EPSs decrease plasma cholesterol and triglycerides concentrations and improve cholesterol ratios due to their ability to bind lipids, thereby reducing intestinal absorption by trapping neutral lipids. Because of the inhibition activity on fat absorption, these molecules act as fat scavengers in the digestive tract and remove fat and cholesterol via excretion (Soh et al., 2003; Patel and Prajapati, 2013; Madhuri et al., 2014).

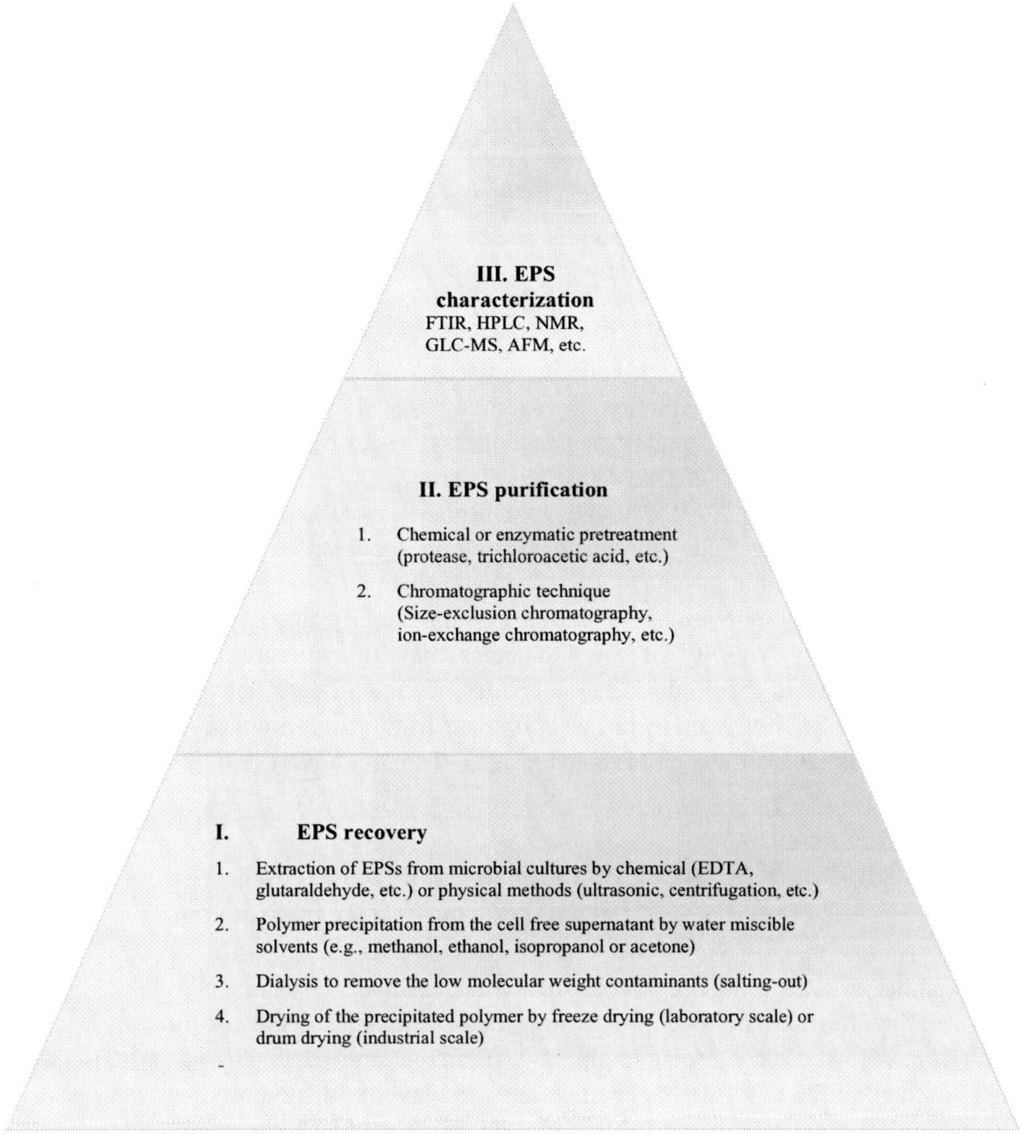

Freitas et al., 2011; Donot et al., 2012; Patel and Prajapati, 2013.

Figure 3. Most steps involved in the recovery, purification and chemical characterization of microbial exopolysaccharides.

Other healthy activities attributed to microbial EPSs include antioxidant, antimicrobial, anti-inflammatory, antidiabetic and anticancer activities (figure 1). Liu et al. (2011) demonstrated that EPSs from *Lactobacillus paracasei* NTU 101 and *L. plantarum* NTU 102 have potential antioxidant properties including *in vitro* 1,1-diphenyl-2-picrylhydrazyl radical scavenging activity, chelation of ferrous ions, inhibition of linoleic acid peroxidation, and reducing power. Orsod et al. (2012) and Mahendran et al. (2013) reported that EPSs extracted from both bacteria and fungi have good potential antimicrobial activities. Ebosin is a novel exopolysaccharide (EPS) produced by *Streptomyces* sp. 139 and evidenced to possess an anti-rheumatic arthritis activity in vivo (Yang et al., 2014).

EPSs produced by *Trichoderma erinaceum* DG-312 was shown to have a strong antiinflammatory activity in inflamed mice (Joo and Yun, 2005). *Enterobacter cloacae* was also found to produce EPSs with anti-diabetic activity (Jin et al., 2012). Many microbial EPSs have an anticancer activity. In general, the action mechanism is via macrophage activation in the host (Im et al., 2010). Chabot et al. (2001) reported that EPSs from *Lactobacillus rhamnosus* RW-9595M stimulate TNF, IL-6 and IL-12 in human and mouse cultured immunocompetent cells, and IFN-gamma in mouse splenocytes. Recently, Matsuda et al. (2003) reported that a sulphated exopolysaccharide produced by Pseudomonas sp. shows a cytotoxic effect towards human cancer cell lines such as MT-4. These findings have resulted in further interest in this polysaccharide as a new anticancer drug suitable for clinical trials.

In addition to associated health benefits, incorporation of the dietary fiber EPSs to food products imparts a number of functional properties to the finished foods, including increased water holding, gel forming, emulsifying, stabilizing, texurizing, and thickening capacities (figure 1) (Smelcerovic et al., 2008; Freitas et al., 2011; Patel and Prajapati, 2013; Tabibloghmany and Ehsandoost, 2014). These properties are important for the organoleptic quality of food products and for their appealing appearance and pleasant mouthfeel. Functional properties of microbial EPSs depend principally on intrinsic physicochemical characteristics such as monosaccharide composition, molecular mass, charge, presence of side chains, polydispersity, rigidity of the molecules and 3D-structures of the polymers. In addition to physical and rheological characteristics, the interactions between EPS and various components in foods contribute to the development of the final product (Smelcerovic et al., 2008; Freitas et al., 2011; Patel and Prajapati, 2013; Tabibloghmany and Ehsandoost, 2014).

VII. Applications of Microbial Exopolysaccharides in Food Industry

A number of microbial polysaccharides (e.g., xanthan, curdlan, pullulan.) have found commercial applications in food processing, replacing some of the traditionally used plant gums (Kumar et al., 2007; Venugopal, 2011; Banerjee and Bhattacharya, 2012). They are usually used as additives to modify the rheology and texture of food products at levels as low as 1 to 3% of formulation weight (Nitta and Nishinari, 2005; Girard and Schaffer-Lequart, 2006; Patel and Prajapati, 2013). Types of such products include dairy products, bakery fillings, confections, dessert gels, icings, jams and jellies and structured foods (figure 1).

Actually, the EPSs produced by lactic acid bacteria (LAB, generally recognised as safe) as kefiran, dextran, alternant, inulin, levan, fructan and reuteran, represent the most suitable polymers for the dairy industry (Duboc and Mollet, 2001; Tsuda, 2013; Madhuri et al., 2014). They are widely employed to improve the texture of fermented dairy products and also to confer health benefits as a result of their immunostimulatory, antitumoral or cholesterol lowering activity (Soccol, et al., 2010). The use of EPS producing starter cultures for yogurt elaboration enhance water retention, texture and confer thickness without altering the organoleptic characteristics of the final product. In the cheese making process strains such as *L.delbrueckii ssp. bulgaricus*, *L. helveticus* and *L. casei*, produce HePS. Their role in cheese production depends on associations with other strains and also on the presence or absence of charges in the EPS produced (Girard and Schaffer-Lequart 2006; Tabibloghmany and

Ehsandoost., 2014). In low-fat dairy products, such as fresh cheese, cream cheese, or processed cheese, the addition of a few percent of EPSs like inulin gives a creamier mouthfeel and imparts a better-balanced round flavor (Stephen et al., 2006). Besides yoghurt and cheeses, other fermented milk products in which EPS-producing cultures have been shown to affect product's rheology are sour cream, and kefir (Patel and Prajapati, 2013).

Microbial EPSs can be used as baking improvers to enhance dough rheological properties and bread quality. Indeed, EPSs have positive effects on water holding capacity and emulsion stability of bread dough. Alginate, levan, dextran, reuteran and other EPSs improve the properties of bread in terms of specific volume index, width/height ratio, crumb hardness, sensory properties (visual appearance, aroma, flavor, crunchiness), and overall acceptability (Brownlee et al., 2005; Arendt et al., 2007; Galle, et al., 2012).

The benefits of microbial EPSs as an additive in muscle products include control of flavor loss, antimicrobial, antioxidant and texturizing properties, and increased storage stability. Storage studies indicated that the coating significantly improved overall appearance and color, juiciness, flavor, texture, and overall palatability of the product. The growth of microorganisms in the product was also removed by the coating (Venugopal, 2011).

Microbial EPSs can be useful for the clarification of a variety of wines and vinegars. Browning and overoxidation are the most common defects in these products (Venugopal, 2011). Reducing their phenolic compounds by the use of EPSs as adsorbents could be an efficient solution to counter these problems. Spagna et al. (1996) reported that chitosan has a high affinity to a number of phenolic compounds, particularly cinnamic acid, and prevents browning in a variety of white wines. It compared well with two conventional adsorbents being used for these applications.

A number of benefits, particularly antioxidant and antimicrobial activities, can be derived from microbial EPSs with regard to fruits and vegetables. These activities are achieved by dipping food products in a solution of EPSs to coat them.

For better antimicrobial activity, the treated products may be stored under modified atmosphere and at chilled temperatures. The microbiological loads on the EPS-coated samples are usually lower in comparison with uncoated products, and the effect depends on the type of fruit and vegetables (Venugopal, 2011; Majolagbe et al., 2013; Zhang et al., 2013). Chitosan added to pickled vegetables inhibits the growth of molds.

A combination of chitosan and highpressure treatment has been recently shown to enhance the storage life of apple juice and apple cider (Venugopal, 2011).

Microbial EPSs belong also to a group of ingredients commonly used in ice cream formulations in order to increase mix viscosity, to stabilize the mix by avoiding crystallisation and shrinkage.

Also, EPSs secure heat shock resistance and allow homogenous melting without whey separation and produce smoothness in texture during consumption (Regand and Goff, 2002). Microbial EPSs such as xanthane, gellan and pullulan have been exploited as materials for the encapsulation of food ingredients (Venugopal, 2011).

Many findings indicate that xanthan, gellan and mixtures of both gums are adequate for the encapsulation of probiotic bacteria greatly improving their survival when exposed to acidic conditions and bile salts (Ding and Shah, 2009).

Conclusion

A vast number of microbial EPSs have been reported over recent years, and their biosynthesis, composition and structural characteristics have been extensively studied. The microbial EPSs have unique functional and rheological properties because of their gelling capacities at low concentrations and their pseudoplastic nature. These interested biomolecules show various technological properties and can be used as biothickeners, texturizers, emulsifiers and foaming stabilizers. The healthy benefits of EPSs encourage also their explorations in food industry. Indeed, these EPSs have been considered as novel dietary fibers and biological response modifiers due to their ability to reduce intestinal absorption and to enhance the immune system and, therefore, prevent several common diseases and promote health. Cancer, cardiovascular diseases, and viral and bacterial infections are among the most studied healthy problems treated with microbial EPSs. In this context, considerable progress has been made in discovering and developing new properties of microbial EPSs. The major limitation of the applications of some of these microbial EPSs has been largely due to cost of production relative to their commercial value; however several approaches have been employed to address these issues such as the optimization of fermentation process by response surface methodology and using cheaper substrates, or the development of higher yielding strains via mutagenesis or genetic and metabolic manipulations. Structure-function studies of microbial EPSs particularly from lactic acid bacteria (GRAS microorganisms) could open the way for enormous research in the field of structural modification and novel food applications.

References

Amjres, H., Béjar, V., Quesada, E., Carranza, D., Abrini, J., Sinquine, C., Ratiskol, J., Colliec-Jouault, S., and Liamas, I. (2015). Characterization of haloglycan, an exopolysaccharide produced by *Halomonas stenophila* HK30. *International Journal of Biological Macromolecules,* 72: 117-124.

Annarita, P. Paola, Di D. Gennaro, R. A. and Barbara, N. (2011). Synthesis, Production, and Biotechnological Applications of Exopolysaccharides and Polyhydroxyalkanoates, *Archaea*, ID 693253, 1-13 doi:10.1155/2011/693253.

Arena, A., Maugeri, T. L., Pavone, B., Iannello, D., Gugliandolo, C., Bisignano, G. (2006). Antiviral and immunoregulatory effect of a novel exopolysaccharide from a marine thermotolerant *Bacillus licheniformis. Int. Immunopharmacol.*, 6: 8-13.

Arena, A., Gugliandolo, C., Stassi, G., Pavone, B., Iannello, D., Bisignano, G., and Maugeri, T. L. (2009). An exopolysaccharide produced by *Geobacillus thermodenitrificans* strain B3-72: Antiviral activity on immunocompetent cells. *Immunol. Lett.*, 123: 132-137.

Arendt, E. K., Ryan, L. A. M. and Dal Bello, F. (2007). Impact of sourdough on the texture of bread. *Food Microbiology*, 24: 165-174.

Banerjee, S. and Bhattacharya, S. (2012). Food Gels: Gelling Process and New Applications, *Food Science and Nutrition*, 52: 334-346.

Boeriu, C. G., Springer, J., Kooy, F. K., van den Broek, L. A. M., and Eggink, G. (2013). Production Methods for Hyaluronan. *International Journal of Carbohydrate Chemistry*, http://dx.doi.org/10.1155/2013/624967.

Brownlee, I. A., Allen, A., Pearson, J. P., Dettmar, P. W., Havler, M. E., Atherton, M. R., and Onnsoyen, E. (2005). Alginate as a Source of Dietary Fiber, *Food Sci. Nutr.* 45: 497-510.

Carrion, O., Delgado, L. and Mercade, E., (2014).New emulsifying and cryoprotective exopolysaccharide from Antarctic *Pseudomonas sp.* ID1. *Carbohydrate Polymers*, http:// dx.doi.org/10.1016/j.carbpol.

Chabot, S., Yu, H. L., De Leseleuc, L., Cloutier, D., van Calsteren, M. R., et al. (2001). Exopolysaccharides from *LactoBacillus rhamnosus* RW-9595M stimulate TNF, IL-6 and IL-12 in human and mouse cultured immunocompetent cells, and IFN-gamma in mouse splenocytes. *Lait* 81: 683-697.

Chung, P. C. K. (2000). Evaluation of mushroom fiber as an alternative source of food fiber. *Supplements in the proceeding from the first international conference on dietary fiber*, Dublin, Ireland, May 13-18, 2000.

Colliec-Jouault, S., Zanchetta, P., Helley, D., Ratiskol, J., Sinquin, C., Fischer, A. M., and Guezennec, J. (2004). Microbial polysaccharides of marine origin and their potential in human therapeutics. *Pathol. Biol.*, 52: 127-130.

Czaczyk, K., Myszka, K. (2007). Biosynthesis of Extracellular Polymeric Substances (EPS) and Its Role in Microbial Biofilm Formation, *Polish J. of Environ. Stud.* 16: 799-806.

Ding, W.-K. and Shah, N.-P.(2009). Effect of various encapsulating materials on the stability of probiotic bacteria. *J. Food Sci.*, 74:100-107.

Donot, F., Fontana, A., Baccou, J. C., and Schorr-Galindo, S. (2012). Microbial exopolysaccharides: Main examples of synthesis, excretion, genetics and extraction. *Carbohydrate Polymers*, 87: 951-962.

De Oliveira, M.-R., da Silva, R.-S.-S.-F., Buzato, J. B., and Celligoi, M.-A.-P.-C. (2007). Study of levan production by *Zymomonas mobilis* using regional low-cost carbohydrate sources. *Biochemical Engineering Journal*, 37: 177-183.

De Vuyst, L. and Degeest, B. (1999). Heteropolysaccharides from lactic acid bacteria, *FEMS Microbiology Reviews* 23: 153-177.

Duboc, P. and Mollet, B. (2001). Applications of exopolysaccharides in the dairy industry. *International Dairy Journal*, 11: 759-768.

Elisashvili, V.-I., Kachlishvili, E.-T., Wasser, S.-P. (2009). Carbon and nitrogen source effects on basidiomycetes exopolysaccharide production. *Appl. Biochem. Micro.+*, 45: 531-5.

Elizaquivel, P., Sanchez, G., Salvador, A., Fiszman, S., Duenas, M. T., Lopez, P., Fernendez de Palencia, P., and Aznar, R. (2011). Evaluation of yogurt and various beverages as carriers of lactic acid bacteria producing 2-branched (1,3)-β-d-glucan. *Journal of Dairy Science*, 94: 3271-3278.

Finore, I., Di Donato, P., Mastascusa, V., Nicolaus, B., and Poli, A. (2014). Fermentation Technologies for the Optimization of Marine Microbial Exopolysaccharide Production, *Mar. Drugs,* 12: 3005-3024.

Freitas, F., Alves, V.-D. and Reis, M.-A.-M. (2011). Advances in bacterial exopolysaccharides: from production to biotechnological applications. *Trends in Biotechnology,* 29: 388-398.

Galle, S., Schwab, C., Dal Bello, F., Michael, A.-C., Gänzle, G., Arendt, E.-K. (2012). Influence of *in-situ* synthesized exopolysaccharides on the quality of gluten-free sorghum sourdough bread, *International Journal of Food Microbiology*, 155: 105-112.

Ganzle, M. and Schwab, C. (2009). Ecology of exopolysaccharide formation by lactic acid bacteria: sucrose utilisation, stress tolerance, and biofilm formation, In: *Bacterial Polysaccharides: Current Innovations and Future Trends,* Matthias Ullrich, pp. (263-278) Caister Academic Press, ISBN 978-1-904455-45-5, Norfolk, UK.

Girard, M. and Schaffer-Lequart, C. (2006). Attractive interactions between selected anionic exopolysaccharides and milk proteins, *Food hydrocoll*, 22:1425.

He, P., Geng, L., Mao, D., and Xu, C. (2012). Production, characterization and antioxidant activity of exopolysaccharides from submerged culture of *Morchella crassipes*. *Bioprocess Biosyst. Eng*. 35:1325-32.

Hwang, J.-W., Yang, Y.-K., Hwang, J.-K., Pyun, Y.-R., and Kim, Y.-S. (1999). Effects of pH and dissolved oxygen on cellulose production by *Acetobacter xylinum* BRC5 in agitated culture. *Bioscience and Bioengineering*, 88: 183-189.

Im, S.-A., Wang, W., Lee, C.-K., and Lee, Y.-N. (2010). Activation of Macrophages by Exopolysaccharide Produced by MK1 Bacterial Strain Isolated from Neungee Mushroom, *Sarcodon aspratus, Immune Netw.*, 10: 230-238.

Jin, M., Lu, Z., Huang, M., and Wang, Y. (2012). Effects of Se - enriched polysaccharide produced by Enterobacter cloacae Z0206 on alloxan-induced diabetic mice. *Int. J. Biol. Macromol*., 50:348-352.

Joo, J.-H. and Yun, J.-W. (2005). Structure and molecular characterization of extracellular polysaccharides produced by Trichoderma erinaceum DG-312. *J. Mol. Biotechnol*., 15: 1250-1257.

Kalogiannis, S., Iakovidou, G., Liakopoulou-Kyriakides, M., Kyriakidis, D.-A., and Skaracis, G.-N. (2003). Optimization of xanthan gum production by *Xanthomonas campestris* grown in molasses. *Process Biochemistry*, 39: 249-256.

Kambourova, M., Mandeva, R., Dimova, D., Poli, A., Nicolaus, B., and Tommonaro, G., (2009). "Production and characterization of a microbial glucan, synthesized by *Geobacillus tepidamans* V264 isolated from Bulgarian hot spring," *Carbohydrate Polymers*, 77: 338-343.

Kumar, A.-S., Mody, K. and Jha, B. (2007). Bacterial exopolysaccharides: a perception. *Journal of Basic Microbiology* 47: 103-117.

Kumari, M., Survase, S.-A. and Singhal, R.-S. (2008). Production of schizophyllan using Schizophyllum commune NRCM. *Bioresource Technology*, 99: 1036-1043.

Lim, J.-M., Kim, S.-W., Hwang, H.-J., et al. (2004) Optimization of medium by orthogonal matrix method for submerged mecelial culture and exopolysaccharide production in *Collybia maculate*. *Appl. Biochem. Biotech*. 119: 159-70.

Lin, M.-H., Yang, Y.-L., Chen, Y.-P., Hua, K.-F., Lu, C.-P., Sheu, F., Lin, G.-H., Tsay, S.-S., Liang, S.-M., and Wu, S.-H. (2011). Novel Exopolysaccharide from the Biofilm of Thermus aquaticus YT-1 Induces the Immune Response through Toll-like Receptor. *J. Biol. Chem*. 286: 17736-17745.

Luo, J., Liu, J., Ke, C., et al. (2009). Optimization of medium composition for the production of exopolysaccharides from *Phellinus baumii* Pilát in submerged culture and the immuno-stimulating activity of exopolysaccharides. *Carbohyd. Polym*.78:409-15.

Liu, C.-F., Tseng, K.-C., Chiang, S.-S., Lee, B.-H., Hsu, W.-H., et al. (2011) Immunomodulatory and antioxidant potential of *Lactobacillus* exopolysaccharides. *J. Sci. Food Agric*. 91: 2284-2291.

Madhuri, K.-V., Prabhakar, K.-V. (2014). Microbial Exopolysaccharides: Biosynthesis and Potential Applications. *Orient. J. Chem.*; 30(3).

Mahapatra, S. and Banerjee, D. (2013). Fungal Exopolysaccharide: Production, Composition and Applications. *Microbiology Insights*: 61-16.

Mahendran, S., Saravanan, S., Vijayabaskar, P., Anandapandian, K.-T.-K., and Shankar, T. (2013). antibacterial potential of microbial exopolysaccharide from *ganoderma lucidum* and lysinibacillus *fusiformis, International Journal of Recent Scientific Research*. 4: 501-505.

Majolagbe, O.-N., Oloke, J.-K., Adebayo, E.-A., Adewoyin, A.-G., Ayandele, A., and Bamigboye, C.-O. (2013). Study on the Antibacterial Activity of Exopolysaccharides of *Lentinus subnudus* Using Swiss Albino Rats as Animal Model. *American-Eurasian Journal of Scientific Research*. 8: 47-52.

Mancuso-Nichols, C.-A., Garon, S., Bowman, J.-P., Raguénès, G., and Guézennec, J. (2004). Production of exopolysaccharides by Antarctic marine bacterial isolates. *J. Appl. Microbiol.,* 96: 1057-1066.

Mann, J. I. and Cummings, J. H. (2009). Possible implications for health of the different definitions of dietary fibre. *Nutrition, Metabolism and Cardiovascular Diseases*, 19: 226-229.

Martensson, O., Duenas-Chasco, M., Irastorza, A., Oste, R., and Holst, O. (2003). Comparison of growth characteristics and exopolysaccharide formation of two lactic acid bacteria strains, *Pediococcus damnosus* 2.6 and Lactobacillus brevis G-77, in an oat-based, nondairy medium. *Lebensm.-Wiss. U.-Technol*., 36: 353-357.

Mata, J.-A., Béjar, V., Liamas, I., Arias, S., Bressollier, P., Tallon, R., Urdaci, M.-C., and Quesada, E. (2006). Exopolysaccharides produced by the recently described halophilic bacteria *Halomonas ventosae* and *Halomonas anticariensis. Research in Microbiology*, 157: 827-835.

Matsuda, M., Yamori, T., Naitoh, M., Okutani, K. (2003). Structural revision of sulfated polysaccharide B-1 isolated from a marine *pseudomonas species* and its cytotoxic activity against human cancer cell lines. *Mar. Biotechnol.* 5: 13-19.

Mcintosh, M., Stone, B.-A., Stanisich, V.-A. (2005). "Curdlan and other bacterial (1-3)-beta-D-glucans". *Appl. Microbiol. Biotechnol.* 68 (2): 163-73.

Mehta, A., Sidhu, C., Pinnaka, A.-K., Roy CèA. (2014). Extracellular Polysaccharide Production by a Novel Osmotolerant Marine Strain of Alteromonas macleodii and Its Application towards Biomineralization of Silver. *PLoS ONE* 9: e98798. doi:10.1371/ journal.pone.0098798.

Mejía, M.-Á., Segura, D., Espín, G., Galindo, E., and Peña, C. (2010). Two-stage fermentation process for alginate production by Azotobacter vinelandii mutant altered in poly-β-hydroxybutyrate (PHB) synthesis. *Journal of Applied Microbiology*, 108: 55-61.

Mozzi, F., Vaningelgem, F., Hebert, E.-M., Van der Meulen, R., Foulquie Moreno, M.-R., Font de Valdez, G., and De Vuyst, L. (2006). Diversity of heteropolysaccharide-producing lactic acid bacterium strains and their biopolymers. *Applied and Environmental Microbiology,* 72: 4431-4435.

Nampoothiri, K.-M., Singhania, R.-R., Sabarinath, C., and Pandey, A. (2003). Fermentative production of gellan using *Sphingomonas paucimobilis*. *Process Biochemistry*, 38: 1513-1519.

Nicolaus, B., Kambourova, M. and Oner, E.-T. (2010). "Exopolysaccharides from extremophiles: from fundamentals to biotechnology,"*Environmental Technology*, 31: 1145-1158.

Nitta, Y. and Nishinari, K. (2005). Gelation and gel properties of polysaccharides gellan gum and tamarind xyloglucan, *J. Biol. Macromol.*, 5: 47-52.

Nwodo, U.-U., Green, E. and Okoh, A.-I. (2012). Bacterial Exopolysaccharides: Functionality and Prospects. *Int. J. Mol. Sci.*, 13: 14002-14015.

Orsod, M., Joseph, M. and Huyop, F. (2012) Characterization of Exopolysaccharides Produced by *Bacillus cereus* and *Brachybacterium* sp. Isolated from Asian Sea Bass (*Lates calcarifer*), *Malaysian Journal of Microbiology*, 8: 170-174.

Parolis, H., Parolis, L.-A.-S., Boán, I.-F., Rodríguez-Valera, F., Widmalm, G., Manca, Mc., Jansson, P.-E., and Sutherland, I.-W. (1993). The structure of the exopolysaccharide produced by the halophilic Archaeon *Haloferax mediterranei* strain R4 (ATCC 33500). *Carbohydr. Res.*, 295: 147-156.

Patel, A. and Prajapati, J.-B. (2013). Food and Health Applications of Exopolysaccharides produced by Lactic acid Bacteria. *Adv. Dairy Res.*, 1:107. doi: 10.4172/2329-888X.10001 07.

Pavlova, K., Koleva, L., Kratchanova, M., and Panchev, I. (2004). Production and characterization of an exopolysaccharide by yeast. *World Journal of Microbiology and Biotechnology*, 20: 435-439.

Pavlova, K., Panchev, I. and Hristozova, T. (2005). Physico-chemical characterization of exomannan from Rhodotorula acheniorum MC. *World Journal of Microbiology and Biotechnology*, 21: 279-283.

Poli, A., Di Donato, P., Abbamondi, G. R., and Nicolaus, B. (2011). Synthesis, Production, and Biotechnological Applications of Exopolysaccharides and Polyhydroxyalkanoates by Archaea (2011). *Hindawi Publishing Corporation Archaea*, 2011: 1-3.

Poli, A., Esposito, E., Orlando, P., Lama, L., Giordano, A., De Appolonia, F., Nicolaus, B., Gambacorta, A. (2007). Halomonas alkaliantarctica sp. nov., isolated from saline lake Cape Russell in Antarctica, an alkalophilic moderately halophilic, exopolysaccharide-producing bacterium. *Syst. Appl. Microbiol.*, 30: 31-38.

Poli, A., Kazak, H., Gurleyendag, B., et al., (2009). High level synthesis of levan by a novel *Halomonas* species growing on defined media. *Carbohydrate Polymers*, 78: 651-657.

Poli, A., Schiano Moriello, V., Esposito, E., Lama, L., Gambacorta, A., and Nicolaus, B. (2004). Exopolysaccharide production by a new Halomonas strain CRSS isolated from saline lake Cape Russell in Antarctica growing on complex and defined media. *Biotechnol. Lett.*, 26: 1635-1638.

Qiang, L., Yumei, L., Sheng, H., Yingzi, L., Dongxue, S., Dake, H., Jiajia, W., Yanhong, Q., Yuxia, Z. (2013). Optimization of Fermentation Conditions and Properties of an Exopolysaccharide from *Klebsiella* sp. H-207 and Application in Adsorption of Hexavalent Chromium. *PLoS One*, 8: e53542.

Ramberg, J.-E., Nelson, E.-D., Sinnott, R.-A. (2010). Immunomodulatory dietary polysaccharides: a systematic review of the literature. *Nutr. J.* 9:1-60.

Ravella, S.-R., Quinones, T.-S.-R., Retter, A., Heiermann, M., Amon, T., and Hobbs, P. J. (2010). Extracellular polysaccharide (EPS) production by a novel strain of yeast-like fungus Aureobasidium pullulans. *Carbohydrate Polymers*, 82: 728-732.

Regand, A. and Goff, H. D. (2002). Effect of Biopolymers on Structure and Ice Recrystallization in Dynamically Frozen Ice Cream Model Systems, *J. Dairy Sci.* 85: 2722-2732.

Rehm, B.-H.-A. (ed.) (2009). *Microbial production of biopolymers and polymer precursors: applications and perspectives,* Caister Academic Press.

Rinker, K.-D. and Kelly, R.-M. (2000). Effect of carbon and nitrogen sources on growth dynamics and exopolysaccharide production for the hyperthermophilic archaeon *Thermococcus litoralis* and bacterium *Thermotoga maritime. Biotechnology and Bioengineering*, 69: 537-547.

Ruas-Madiedo, P., Hugenholtz, J., Zoon, P. (2002). An overview of the functionality of exopolysaccharides produced by lactic acid bacteria. *Int. Dairy J.* 12:163-171.

Shih, I.-L., Chen, L.-D. and Wu, J.-Y. (2010). Levan production using *Bacillus subtilis* natto cells immobilized on alginate. *Carbohydrate Polymers*, 82: 111-117.

Shih, I.-L., Yu, J.-Y., Hsieh, C., and Wu, J.-Y. (2009). Production and characterization of curdlan by *Agrobacterium sp. Biochemical Engineering Journal*, 43: 33-40.

Singha, T.-K. (2012). Microbial Extracellular Polymeric Substances: Production, Isolation and Applications, *IOSR Journal of Pharmacy*, 2: 276-281.

Smelcerovic, A., Knezevic-Jugovic, Z. and Petronijevic, Z. (2008). Microbial Polysaccharides and their Derivatives as Current and Prospective Pharmaceuticals. *Current Pharmaceutical Design*, 14, 000-000.

Soccol, C.-R., De Souza, L.-P., Vandenberghe, M.-R., Spier, A.-B., Pedroni Medeiros, C., Yamaguishi, T., J. De D. Lindner, Pandey, A., and Thomaz-Soccoll, V. (2010). The Potential of Probiotics: A Review. *Food Technol. Biotechnol.* 48: 413-434.

Soh, H.-S., Kim, C.-S., Lee, S.-P. (2003). A New *In vitro* Assay of Cholesterol Adsorption by Food and Microbial Polysaccharides. *J. Med. Food* 6: 225-230.

Spagna, G., et al., (1996). The stabilization of white wines by absorption of phenolic compounds on chitin and chitosan, *Food Res. Int.* 29: 241.

Stephen, A.-M., Phillips, G.-O., Williams, P.-A. (2006). *Food Polysaccharides and Their Applications*, Taylor and Francis Group, LLC, 335-349.

Stredansky, M. and Conti, E. (1999). Succinoglycan production by solid-state fermentation with *Agrobacterium tumefaciens. Applied microbiology and biotechnology*, 52: 332-7.

Streit, F., Koch, F., Laranjeira, M.-C.-M., and Ninow, J. L. (2009). Production of fungal chitosan in liquid cultivation using apple pomace as substrate. *Braz. J. Microbiol.*, 40: 20-25.

Survase, S.-A., Saudagar, P.-S. and Singhal, R.-S. (2007). Use of complex media for the production of scleroglucan by *Sclerotium rolfsii* MTCC 2156. *Bioresource Technol.*, 98: 1509-1512.

Tabibloghmany, F.-S. and Ehsandoost, E. (2014). An Overview of Healthy and Functionality of Exopolysacharides Produced by Lactic Acid Bacteria in the Dairy Industry. *European Journal of Nutrition and Food Safety*, 4: 63-86.

Tapan, K.-S. (2012). Microbial Extracellular Polymeric Substances: Production, Isolation and applications, *IOSR Journal of Pharmacy*, 2: 276-281.

Tavares, A. P. M., Agapito, M. S. M., Coelho, M. A. Z., et al. (2005). Selection and optimization of culture medium for exopolysaccharide production by *Coriolus (Trametes) versicolor*. *World J. Microb. Biot.*, 21:1499-507.

Tok, E., Aslim, B. (2010). Cholesterol removal by some lactic acid bacteria that can be used as probiotic. *Microbiol. Immunol.* 54: 257-264.

Tsuda, H. (2013). Exopolysaccharides of Lactic Acid Bacteria for food and Colon health applications, In: Marcelino, K. *Lactic Acid Bacteria - R and D for Food, Health and Livestock Purposes, In Tech*, 517-538.

Vedyashkina, T.-A., Revin, V.-V. and Gogotov, I.-N. (2005). Optimizing the conditions of dextran synthesis by the bacterium *Leuconostoc mesenteroides* grown in a molasses-containing medium. *Appl. Biochem. Microbiol.*, 41:361-364.

Venugopal, V. (2011). *Marine Polysaccharides: Food Applications*, Taylor and Francis Group, LLC.

Werning, M.-L., Notararigo, S., Nácher, M., De Palencia, P.-F., Aznar, R., and López, P. (2012). *Biosynthesis, Purification and Biotechnological Use of Exopolysaccharides Produced by Lactic Acid Bacteria, Food Additive,* Prof. Yehia El-Samragy (Ed.), ISBN: 978-953-51-0067-6, InTech.

Wu, J., Zhan, X., Liu, H., and Zheng, Z. (2008). Enhanced production of curdlan by *Alcaligenes faecalis* by Selective feeding with ammonia water during the cell growth phase of fermentation. *Chinese Journal of Biotechnology*, 24: 1035-1039.

Xu, C.-P., Kim, S.-W., Hwang, H.-J., Choi, J.-W., and Yun, J.-W. (2003). Optimization of submerged culture conditions for mycelial growth and exo-biopolymer production by *Paecilomyces tenuipes* C240. *Process Biochem*. 38:1025-30.

Yang, H. and He, G. (2008). Influence of nutritional conditions on exopolysaccharide production by submerged cultivation of the medicinal fungus *Shiraia bambusicola*. *World J. Microb. Biot*. 24: 2903-7.

Yang, Z., Junjie, S., Yonggang, B., Liping, B., Rong, J., Lianhong, G., Chen, Y., Ren, Z., and Yuan, L. (2014). Characterization of an Ebosin derivative produced by heterologous gene replacement in Streptomyces sp. 139, *Microbial Cell Factories*, 13:103.

Zhang, B.-B. and Cheung, C.-K. (2011). Use of stimulatory agents to enhance the production of bioactive exopolysaccharide from *Pleurotus tuber-regium* by submerged fermentation. *J. Agr. Food Chem*. 59:1210-6.

Zhang, J., Wang, R., Jiang, P., Lui, Z. (2002). Production of an exopolysaccharide bioflocculant by *Sorangium cellulosum*. *Lett. Appl. Microbiol*. 34:178-81.

Zhang, L., Liu, C., Li, D., Zhao, Y., Zhang, X., Zeng, X., Yang, Z., and Li, S. (2013). Antioxidant activity of an exopolysaccharide isolated from *Lactobacillus plantarum* C88. *Int. J. Biol. Macromol.* 54: 270-275.

Zhang, Y.-Z. (2011). Optimization of Fermentation Conditions and Rheological Properties of Exopolysaccharide Produced by Deep-Sea Bacterium *Zunongwangia profunda* SM-A87. *PLoS One*, *6*: e26825.

INDEX

A

B

C

D

E

F

G

H

I

K

L

M

N

O

P

Q

R

S

T

U

V

W

X

Y

Z